FOR THOSE AT RISK . . .

This book is for you and your loved ones! It includes information from the Third Report of the National Cholesterol Education Program Expert Panel on Detection, Evaluation and Treatment of High Blood Cholesterol in Adults. A chapter on cholesterol concerns of children and adolescents is included.

Anyone, regardless of age, gender or ethnic background, can develop a blood cholesterol problem without even being aware of it. Are you one of the many individuals who has or is at risk for developing cardiovascular disease? Why chance the risk of heart disease, stroke or other vascular problems?

This book:

- Enables you to understand and work more easily with your physician in controlling your blood cholesterol.
- Is a guide for having your cholesterol levels checked and helping you understand the results.
- Enables you to discover your risk of developing coronary heart disease and deal with the resolution.
- Enables you to be successful in controlling your cholesterol levels, if necessary, in the easiest way and the shortest period of time.
- Helps you understand some basic information about your body chemistry and its relationship to the foods you eat and their relationship to blood cholesterol.
- Explains the relationship of cholesterol to cardiovascular diseases.

Cholesterol control is a personal experience. Only through personal initiative, understanding your body chemistry and following a correct program can you control your cholesterol.

The information in this book is not for self diagnosing but does enable you to work more effectively with your doctor. Physicians recommend this book.

Note: Children should not be placed on a low fat, low cholesterol diet unless prescribed by their physician. Children in their early years require a moderate amount of fat for proper development.

SAVE YOUR LIFE!

Every minute of every day:
   One American experiences his/her first stroke
   Three Americans have heart attacks
   One American dies from a heart attack

Think about it!

Controlling your cholesterol is the foremost thing you can do to help your heart and vascular system be healthy.

This user friendly book tells you all you need to know to control your cholesterol. If you have cholesterol problems or wish to avoid the risk, this is the best book for you.

HERE IS CONCISE INFORMATION IN PLAIN LANGUAGE ABOUT:

- How to control your cholesterol levels
- How to lose and/or control your weight
- Importance of decreasing saturated fat intake
- Choosing the type of exercise to help control your cholesterol
- A 3 week plan for controlling cholesterol
- Food logistics and menus
- How serious high cholesterol is
- How to determine if you have cholesterol problems
- Questions and answers you need to know
- Cholesterol lowering recipes in the cookbook section
- Cholesterol concerns of children and adolescents

The authors give you solutions to the problem.

Controlling your cholesterol levels improves your life and may save it.

REVISED AND UPDATED
A NEW CHAPTER FOR
CHILDREN AND ADOLESCENTS

Cholesterol
C<u>ontrol</u>

3 WEEK PLAN

HANDBOOK and COOKBOOK

Patricia T. Krimmel
Edward A. Krimmel

Preface by
David M. Capuzzi, M.D., Ph.D.

Illustrator,
Art & Design Editor
Charles A. Krimmel

FRANKLIN PUBLISHERS   P.O. Box 1338, Bryn Mawr, PA 19010

AVAILABLE FROM FRANKLIN PUBLISHERS
See order form in back of book

THE LOW BLOOD SUGAR HANDBOOK By *Edward and Patricia Krimmel.*

Highly praised by Harvey Ross, M.D., this is a new upscaled approach to the diagnosis and treatment of hypoglycemia (low blood sugar), written with the insight and practicality that only a sufferer could have, but backed up by meticulous research and medical accuracy. The book of solutions! 192 pages

THE LOW BLOOD SUGAR COOKBOOK By *Patricia and Edward Krimmel.*

A very special collection of over 200 sugarless natural food recipes. Snacks to gourmet dishes designed specifically for the hypoglycemic, but which everyone can enjoy and are also valuable to diabetics and weight watchers. No artificial sweeteners or white flour are used in the recipes. Only fruit and fruit juices are used as sweeteners. 192 pages

THE LOW BLOOD SUGAR CASSETTE By *Patricia and Edward Krimmel.*

A one (1) hour interview conceptualizing many of the most important questions and answers pertaining to hypoglycemia. Receive the feeling of personal contact with the authors.

VITAL HEALTH FACTS and Composition of Foods
By *Edward and Patricia Krimmel*

Aids you in knowing calorie and saturated fat content of foods, your vitamin, mineral and calorie requirements and how to exercise. With this information you can control your weight, fat intake and cholesterol levels all of which lead to better health. Over 100 toll free phone numbers for health information and support.

CHOLESTEROL CONTROL 3 WEEK PLAN: HANDBOOK and COOKBOOK By *Patricia and Edward Krimmel.*

Tells how to be properly tested. Do you know which foods to avoid and why, and which foods to eat and why? Do you want to understand how to lose weight correctly and easily for a lifetime? Do you know which oils to use and which to avoid and how to decrease the amount of saturated fat you eat? Have you taken to task the issue of your child's or adolescent's cholesterol levels? All these issues and many, many more are covered in clear, easy to understand language for a lifetime of benefit. A physician recommend book for vital information and tasty recipes.

ISBN 0-916503-08-9   Printed in the U.S.A.

CONTENTS

PREFACE

By David M. Capuzzi, M.D., Ph.D

Dr. Capuzzi is Director of the Cardiovascular Disease Prevention Center, Director of the Center's Lipoprotein - Atherosclerosis Laboratory, and Professor of Medicine, Biochemistry, and Molecular Pharmacology, Thomas Jefferson University, Philadelphia, Pennsylvania. He is attending Physician in Endocrinology, Diabetes, Metabolism, and Preventive Cardiology at the Thomas Jefferson University Hospital, and Consulting Physician in diabetes and Endocrinology at the Lankenau Hospital, Wynnewood, Pennsylvania. Dr. Capuzzi and his coworkers have conducted many research studies in this field, and have documented their finding in numerous scientific articles.

Over the past decade, since the prior edition of this book, an avalanche of scientific articles have been written describing the new links between blood cholesterol control and cardiovascular disease risk. Novel discoveries have been made on the detection, evaluation, and treatment of blood lipid disorders and related conditions to prevent the occurrence of heart attack and stroke. However, with each new scientific discovery, new issues are raised and prior concepts that seemed settled become open to question. The public understands that something can and should be done to reduce the risk of cardiovascular disease. However, conflicting messages from an array of information sources continue to create uncertainty, skepticism, and often misunderstanding. As a result, a number of questions arise: How can current medical information be translated into practical measures to control blood cholesterol levels? Should these measures be applied to the entire population or only to those at high risk? How should age, sex and other factors be considered in formulating medical evaluation and treatment plans for individuals? How and how often should patients be evaluated to determine their progress and overall health? How can issues of safety, efficacy, expense and inconvenience of various treatment modalities be dealt with in the best interests of the patient? How can the increasing issues of cost containment and for profit influences in the delivery of health care be managed so that prevention of disease is properly emphasized? How can adherence to preventive measures be best maintained over the long term? There are no easy remedies to these questions.

The National Cholesterol Education Program has released its latest recommendations to update both health care professionals and the public about steps that should be taken to lower coronary disease risk. Coronary atherosclerosis is a complex disease caused by an interplay of hereditary and environmental influences. However, through a careful, critical review of the enormous body of available medical evidence, a number of reasoned conclusions can be reached:

- Overwhelming and consistent evidence links high blood cholesterol in a causal fashion with increased risk of premature development of coronary heart disease.
- The higher the blood cholesterol level, the greater the coronary risk.
- Intake of a high cholesterol, high saturated fat, calorie-rich diet is a major contributing factor to high blood cholesterol levels and increased coronary risk.
- Other risk factors such as family history of premature cardiovascular disease, tobacco use, the presence of diabetes mellitus, hypertension, excessive weight, sedentary lifestyle, and stress increase the absolute risk imparted by high blood cholesterol.
- Lowering of elevated blood cholesterol levels by a healthful diet that is low in total calories, saturated fat and high-calorie starches and sugars, but rich in plant fiber along with a prudent, consistent exercise program may contribute to controlling both one's cholesterol and reducing one's vascular risk.
- Judicious use of lipid-lowering medication together with the above therapeutic lifestyle changes (TLC) is very often necessary especially in patients whose cholesterol problem has a strong genetic component.
- Reduction or removal of other modifiable risk factors at any given cholesterol level is a beneficial and necessary part of an optimal treatment plan.

The benefits from blood cholesterol control appear to be greatest in those who are at increased cardiovascular risk for other reasons. However, there is individual variation in response to treatment and there is no unqualified assurance of a health advantage of every individual who undertakes such measures. Therefore, there is no substitute for evaluation by a dedicated physician capable of assessing carefully the cause and risk for blood cholesterol elevation in a given individual. The physician can then decide upon prudent intervention measures, and prescribe a safe, effective regimen to regulate the blood lipids and to reduce or eliminate other modifiable risks to the patient.

There is also a crucial role and responsibility that the patient plays in adhering to the treatment plan. The treatment program should be one that is tailored to and doable by a given patient. Suitable reading material should be provided as a valuable adjunct to a treatment program. In this book, the authors focus on sound basic principles, in a clear and concise format. Sufficient background material is given on cholesterol metabolism and arterial plaque development in a readable, understandable style. The authors have emphasized the importance of utilizing simple tools to reach achievable goals with appropriate health care supervision. This book can supplement the patient's basic knowledge while under the care of a physician, and provide a valuable primer on this subject. The recipes can be utilized or modified to suit personal food preferences and to complement dietary information obtained from a dietician or physician. The updated guidelines for blood cholesterol control provided by the Adult Treatment Panel III of the National Cholesterol Education Program correctly emphasize restricted dietary intake of saturated fat, calories and cholesterol and regular exercise as initial TLC measures to control blood cholesterol level. A diet tailored to suit individual tastes and needs over a long term is essential. The use of medications in addition to lifestyle changes is also addressed by these guidelines. The future holds promise for continued advances in this field and improved therapies. However, a prudent diet remains its cornerstone. The authors have provided an interesting and timely new addition to the available literature in the critical area of cardiovascular risk reduction.

We dedicate this book to:

You, the reader.
Everyone who is interested in his/her well-being.
Those brave people who are willing to think about their body
   chemistry and modify their behavior so they will have more
   healthful and fulfilling lives.
To Helen, Taylor, Rose and George, our Parents, in loving memory of
   their goodness.
The memory of Bob, Al and John.
To all our loved ones.
To the glory of the Lord and may all things be done with the under-
   standing of the Word.

ACKNOWLEDGMENTS

Our special thanks to the individuals who made valuable contributions
to this book, whether by lending an ear, reading the manuscript, making
suggestions or testing recipes. We could never have completed this book
without the help and assistance of Frank Smith, Dr. David Capuzzi,
Charles Krimmel, Dr. Gretchen Krimmel, Dr. Freyda Neyman, Phyllis
McCuen, Charles Foley, Kim Henney, Ron Henney, Dan and Connie
Rondeau, Ethel Young, Lewis and Celia Creskoff, John and Betty
Aukstikalnes, and Shizhe and Hong Zhu.

Take a Chance

There's someone for everyone,
And a place in life too.
You can be anything,
Accept no handicaps,
Settle for nothing but the best.
It's yours for the taking,
Never give up,
Never give in.
Don't let others bring you down,
Strive,
Survive,
And Never be afraid,
To take a chance.

Welcome to: The Essence of Me
Dan G. Smith, Poet, Chula Vista, CA

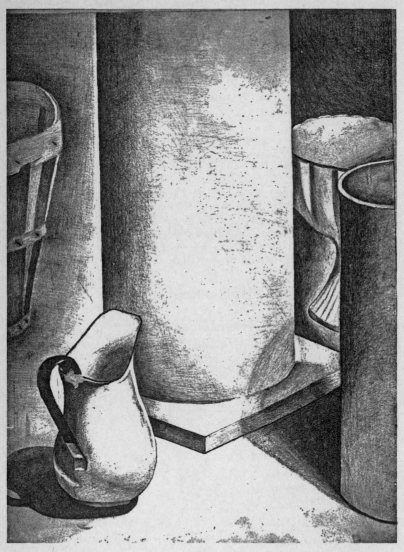

Charles Krimmel

1

UNDERSTANDING CHOLESTEROL

Check your cholesterol and heart disease I.Q.

The following questions and answers were prepared by the National Cholesterol Education Program; National Heart, Lung, and Blood Institute, National Institutes of Health

Are you cholesterol smart? Test your knowledge about high blood cholesterol with the following statements. Circle each true or false. The answers are given at the end of the questions.

1. High blood cholesterol is one of the risk factors for heart disease that you can do something about.
   T   F

2. To lower your blood cholesterol level you must stop eating meat altogether.   T   F

3. Any blood cholesterol level below 240 mg/dL is desirable for adults.   T   F

4. Fish oil supplements are recommended to lower blood cholesterol.   T   F

5. To lower your blood cholesterol level you should eat less saturated fat, total fat, and cholesterol, and lose weight if you are overweight.   T   F

6. Saturated fats raise your blood cholesterol level more than anything else in your diet.   T   F

7. All vegetable oils help lower blood cholesterol levels.
                                                         T   F

8. Lowering blood cholesterol levels can help people who have already had a heart attack.   T   F

9. All children need to have their blood cholesterol levels checked.   T   F

10. Women don't need to worry about high blood cholesterol and heart disease.   T   F

11. Reading food labels can help you eat the heart healthy   way.   T   F

How cholesterol smart are you? Check your answers below.

Answers to the Cholesterol and Heart Disease I.Q. Quiz

1. True. High blood cholesterol is one of the risk factors for heart disease that a person can do something about. High blood pressure, cigarette smoking, diabetes, overweight, and physical inactivity are the others.

2. False. Although some red meat is high in saturated fat and cholesterol, which can raise your blood cholesterol, you do not need to stop eating it or any other single food. Red meat is an important source of protein, iron, and other vitamins and minerals. You should, however, cut back on the amount of saturated fat and cholesterol that you eat. A couple of ways to do this is by choosing lean cuts of meat with the fat trimmed; watch your portion sizes and eat no more than 6 ounces of meat a day. Six ounces is about the size of two decks of playing cards.

3. False. A total blood cholesterol level of under 200 mg/dL is desirable and usually puts you at a lower risk for heart disease. A blood cholesterol level of 240 mg/dL is high and increases your risk of heart disease. If your cholesterol level is high, your doctor will want to check your level of LDL-cholesterol ("bad" cholesterol). A HIGH level of LDL-cholesterol increases your risk of heart disease, as does a LOW level of HDL-cholesterol ("good "cholesterol). An HDL-cholesterol level below 40 mg/dL is considered a risk factor for heart disease. A total cholesterol level of 200-239 mg/dL is considered borderline-high and usually increases your risk for heart disease. All adults 20 years of age or older should have their blood cholesterol level checked at least once every 5 years.

4. False. Fish oils are a source of omega-3 fatty acids, which are a type of polyunsaturated fat. Fish oil supplements generally do not reduce blood cholesterol levels. Also, the effect of the long-term use of fish oil supplements is not known. However, fish is a good food choice because it is low in saturated fat.

5. True. Eating less fat, especially saturated fat, and cholesterol can lower your blood cholesterol level. Generally your blood cholesterol level should begin to drop a few weeks after you start on a cholesterol-lowering diet. How much your level drops depends on the amounts of saturated fat and cholesterol you used to eat, how high your blood cholesterol is, how much weight you lose if you are overweight, and how your body responds to the changes you make. Over time, you may reduce your blood cholesterol level by 10-50 mg/dL or even more.

6. True. Saturated fats raise your blood cholesterol level more than anything else. So, the best way to reduce your cholesterol level is to cut back on the amount of saturated fats that you eat. These fats are found in largest amounts in animal products such as butter, cheese, whole milk, ice cream, cream, and fatty meats. They are also found in some vegetable oils--coconut, palm, and palm kernel oils.

7. False. Most vegetable oils--canola, corn, olive, safflower, soybean, and sunflower oils--contain mostly monounsaturated and polyunsaturated fats, which help lower blood cholesterol when used in place of saturated fats. However, a few vegetable oils-- coconut, palm, and palm kernel oils--contain more saturated fat than unsaturated fat. A special kind of fat, called "trans fat," is formed when vegetable oil is hardened to become margarine or shortening, through a process called "hydrogenation." The harder the margarine or shortening, the more likely it is to contain more trans fat. Choose margarine containing liquid vegetable oil as the first ingredient. Just be sure to limit the total amount of any fats or oils, since even those that are unsaturated are rich sources of calories.

8. True.   People who have had one heart attack are at much higher risk for a second attack. Reducing blood cholesterol levels can greatly slow down (and, in some people, even reverse) the buildup of cholesterol and fat in the wall of the coronary arteries and significantly reduce the chances of a second heart attack. If you have had a heart attack or have coronary heart disease, your LDL level should be around 100 mg/dL which is even lower than the recommended level of less than 130 mg/dL for the general population.

9. False. Children from "high risk" families, in which a parent has high blood cholesterol (240 mg/dL or above) or in which a parent or grandparent has had heart disease at an early age (at 55 years or younger), should have their cholesterol levels tested. If a child from such a family has a cholesterol level that is high, it should be lowered under medical supervision, primarily with diet, to reduce the risk of developing heart disease as an adult. For most children, who are not from high-risk families, the best way to reduce the risk of adult heart disease is to follow a low saturated fat, low cholesterol eating pattern. All children over the age of 2 years and all adults should adopt a heart healthy eating pattern as a principal way of reducing coronary heart disease. (See chapter, Cholesterol Concerns of Children and Adolescent).

10. False. Blood cholesterol levels in both men and women begin to go up around age 20. Women before menopause have levels that are lower than men of the same age. After menopause, a women's LDL-cholesterol level goes up--and so her risk for heart disease increases. For both men and women, heart disease is the number one cause of death.

11. True. Food labels have been changed. Look on the nutrition label for the amount of saturated fat, total fat, cholesterol, and total calories in a serving of the product. Use this information to compare similar products. Also, look for the list of ingredients. Here, the ingredient in the greatest amount is first and the ingredient in the least amount is last. So to choose foods low in saturated fat or total fat, go easy on products that list fats or oil first, or that list many fat and oil ingredients.

If you think the issue of cholesterol is hot and or new, let's just get a few facts from medical history straight and current. As early as 1908, a Russian researcher by the name of Ignatowsky fed rabbits meat, milk and eggs for several months. He discovered that their aortas (largest artery) developed arteriosclerotic lesions. The lesions contained deposits of lipids (fats) and cholesterol and closely resembled the arteriosclerotic lesions found in humans. For the first time, it was shown that arteriosclerosis (a narrowing and clogging of arteries) could be induced by the foods one ate, dispelling the notion that arteriosclerosis had an infectious origin. However Ignatowsky's findings mainly gave rise to another misconception, that arteriosclerosis was a disease caused by protein intoxication.

Another Russian researcher, Anitschkow, thought that the cholesterol in the lesions might have come from the cholesterol in the food the rabbits were fed. He and his associate fed rabbits purified cholesterol and discovered that the rabbits developed high blood cholesterol as well as deposits of lipids and cholesterol in their liver, spleen, arteries and other tissues. The lesions in the arteries contained abundant lipids and cholesterol. From his results, Anitschkow concluded that cholesterol in food could induce arteriosclerosis.

In 1916 the Dutch physician DeLangen believed high blood cholesterol levels increased the incidence of atherosclerosis and gall stones among Javanese people working on Dutch ships. Both of these conditions were rare among native Javanese, but those who ate the meat and dairy foods of the rich Dutch diet developed high blood cholesterol and arteriosclerosis.

Since these early discoveries, much more has been learned about cholesterol. In 1968, research established that the build up of cholesterol in the plaques of arteries comes from the LDL cholesterol in the blood stream.

What may be even more important, additional research has unequivocally shown that eating saturated fat raises blood cholesterol levels more than consuming foods rich in cholesterol but low in saturated fat such as shell fish.

Because research continues, you must keep abreast of the new information available and actively seek it out.

Much of the information in this book comes from the 2001 Third Report of the National Cholesterol Education Program (NCEP) Expert Panel on Detection, Evaluation, and Treatment of High Blood Cholesterol in Adults (Adult Treatment Panel III). This report makes up the NCEP's updated clinical guidelines for cholesterol testing and management. Its major new feature is a focus on primary prevention in persons with multiple risk factors for coronary heart disease (CHD).

Attention!!!
Individuals who have CHD before the age of 55 may have children who have CHD risk factors that need attention. See chapter, Cholesterol Concerns of Children and Adolescents

---

In order for you to grasp the concepts related to blood cholesterol and its relationship to your overall body chemistry, you must do two things:

1. Learn a few new terms and their relationship to your body chemistry.
2. Be patient while trying to learn, understand, and apply the information.

To control your cholesterol, you do not need to learn all of the scientific information related to cholesterol. However, it is sometimes easier to do something if you understand the real reasons for what you are doing. You decide how far you want to delve into the scientific information.

To help you understand the technical terms contained in the text, we give workable definitions of the terms as they occur. Understanding the terms is very important for your being able to learn the concepts which are necessary for your long term progress. We tried to keep the new terms to a minimum.

CHOLESTEROL, A VITAL PART OF YOUR BODY CHEMISTRY

In recent years cholesterol has been under heavy attack. It seems every authority, except for the local dog catcher, has been giving it a bad rap. The truth of the matter is that cholesterol is essential for the cells in your body. However, too much of any good thing can cause serious health problems. Excess cholesterol increases your risk for developing coronary heart disease (CHD) and/or a stroke.

WHAT IS CHOLESTEROL AND WHERE DOES IT COME FROM?

Cholesterol is a soft, odorless, waxy-type substance which is part of all animal cells, including those of humans. It is one of a number of fats, called lipids, found in the blood.

There are two primary sources of cholesterol:
1. From within the body--the liver, intestine and skin produce all the cholesterol the body needs.
2. From foods we eat--foods only of animal origin such as:
   egg yolks
   dairy products
   meats, fish, poultry

The cholesterol content of meat is found mostly in the lean tissue not the fat. A food may contain substantial cholesterol but only a moderate amount of fat (for example, a large egg has only 5gms. of fat but 215 mgs. of cholesterol). Foods of plant origin have no cholesterol.

The amount of cholesterol produced by the body is determined by your body chemistry and possibly by the amount of cholesterol you eat. It may be that for some people, the more cholesterol eaten the less the body produces but this connection has not yet been proven.

WHY DO WE NEED CHOLESTEROL?

Cholesterol is essential to the body's chemistry. Some examples are:

- Is a key substance in the walls of every cell
- Is an aid in hormone production
- Is essential for brain and nerve development
- Is the starting material from which the liver produces bile acids which are necessary for the digestion of fats
- Is the precursor for production of steroid hormones by the adrenal glands and gonads
- Is used to produce Vitamin D

Remember, since your body can manufacture all of the cholesterol it needs, you may not need to consume any additional amounts. It is, however, unnecessary and almost impossible to avoid cholesterol completely.

HOW CHOLESTEROL TRAVELS THROUGH YOUR BODY

Since cholesterol is a fat, it does not mix with water or blood, and cannot travel in the bloodstream by itself. In order for cholesterol and other fats (lipids) to travel through the bloodstream, they must be wrapped in protein. The combination of cholesterol and protein is called "lipoprotein" cholesterol.

The three lipoproteins we will be concerned with are:

1. Very low density lipoprotein (VLDL) cholesterol
2. Low density lipoprotein (LDL) cholesterol
3. High density lipoprotein (HDL) cholesterol

Lipoproteins

Lipoproteins are classified by weight or density of the protein:

- **VLDLs** (Very Low-Density Lipoproteins) carry some cholesterol but mainly triglycerides which the liver produces from excess calories eaten. When the VLDLs travel through the blood stream, the majority of triglycerides are removed to be used as energy or stored as fat. As the process occurs, the VLDLs are gradually converted to LDLs.

- **LDLs** (Low-Density Lipoproteins) carry about 75-80% of the cholesterol in the blood. Cholesterol is transported by the LDLs from the liver to other parts of the body where it can be used for essential functions.

- **HDLs** (High-Density Lipoproteins) carry about 20-25% of the cholesterol in the blood. They transport cholesterol from the body's tissues to the liver where it is eliminated.

Why are LDLs called "bad" cholesterol?

LDLs are the main source of cholesterol buildup and blockage in the arteries. An elevated LDL cholesterol level is a major cause of CHD.

Each cell in your body has receptors which reach out to the LDLs in the blood stream and pull the LDLs into the cell for productive work in cell growth. A diet rich in cholesterol or saturated fats causes fewer receptors for LDLs to be made. If there are too few receptors for the amount of LDLs circulating in the bloodstream, some LDLs will be left in the bloodstream and return to the liver where they will be disposed of. But there will be some that will not be disposed of, and these are the ones that will become stuck on the artery walls and begin the build up of plaque leading to the a narrowing of the opening of the arteries.

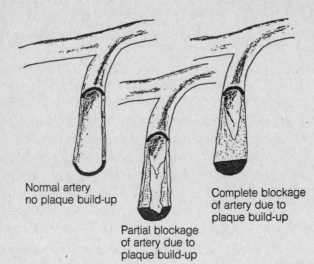

Normal artery
no plaque build-up

Partial blockage
of artery due to
plaque build-up

Complete blockage
of artery due to
plaque build-up

An obvious picture begins to develop. Within the artery walls of a given individual who has too many LDL particles floating around, plaque build up may continue until the opening of the artery becomes so narrow that the blood flow is restricted or stopped completely. It does sound like a pretty good case for calling LDLs "bad".

CHD or a stroke may occur when there is narrowing of the heart arteries because of some significant and dangerous circumstance that may occur such as:

1. The amount of blood carrying the needed supply of oxygen and nutrients to the heart muscle becomes limited resulting in less oxygen and nutrients reaching the heart muscle than it requires to function properly. This can cause angina pectoris (vague ache to severe chest pain and a sensation of constriction about the heart).

2. A blood clot may form due to the plaque buildup and block the blood from reaching the heart muscle reducing the supply of needed oxygen and nutrients causing that area of muscle to be damaged or die.

3. If a blood clot forms, a piece of the blood clot may break off and travel to the brain causing a stroke.

Elevated LDLs are bad, bad, bad! That is why they are your number one target for avoiding CHD and stroke.

Your goal is a low LDL cholesterol level. How this is achieved is discussed in the chapter, How To Control Your Cholesterol.

Cholesterol Numbers
Cholesterol and triglycerides are measured in milligrams per deciliter (mg/dl) and the numbers are usually written with mg/dl after the number (200 mg/dl). For easier reading, we have omitted the mg/dl and stated only the numbers.

Why are HDLs called "good" cholesterol?

HDLs help keep cholesterol from building up in the arteries by carrying cholesterol away from cells in the artery walls back to the liver for reprocessing or removal from the body through the bile acids. Low HDL cholesterol is a strong independent predictor of CHD. Low HDLs is also a risk factor for having a stroke in individuals with CHD. A low level of HDL cholesterol seems to increase the risk of CHD and a high level seems to lower the risk for CHD. Subsequently, HDLs have become known as the "good" guys. Sounds like a good reason to strive for a relatively high level of HDL cholesterol. How to achieve this is explained under the physical activity section in the chapter, How To Control Your Cholesterol.

What Are Triglycerides and What Do They Do?

Triglycerides are fats carried through the blood from the intestines and liver to the body's cells to be used for energy. Triglycerides make up most animal and vegetable fats and comprise the major portion of the fat in your body. Only a small portion of triglycerides are found in the bloodstream.

Excess calories, especially from heavily starchy and heavily sweet carbohydrates, are stored as triglycerides in your fatty tissues.

Recent research indicates that too many triglycerides in the blood stream are an independent risk factor for CHD. High triglycerides is a risk factor for a stroke in individuals with CHD. Therefore you should strive for a low level of triglycerides.

Factors that contribute to elevated triglycerides in the blood of the general population are:

- obesity and overweight
- physical inactivity
- cigarette smoking
- excess alcohol intake
- high carbohydrate diet (> 60% of calories)
- type 2 diabetes
- chronic renal failure
- nephrotic syndrome
- certain drugs - corticosteroids, estrogen, retinoids, higher doses of beta-adrenergic blocking agents

• genetic disorders - familial combined hyperlipidemia, familial hypertriglyceridemia, and familia dysbetalipo- proteinemia

For information on how to lower your triglyceride level, see the chapter How To Control Your Cholesterol.

UNDERSTANDING BLOOD CHOLESTEROL LEVELS

Your blood cholesterol levels play a significant role in your chances of getting CHD. "High blood cholesterol" means that you have more cholesterol present in your bloodstream than is necessary for normal, healthy functioning.

Formerly it was only the total cholesterol level that was looked at in relation to your risk for CHD. Now, because of recent research, all the various types of cholesterol (HDLs, LDLs, VLDLs) and triglycerides are looked at along with various risk factors.

Getting a Focus on Cholesterol and Triglyceride Levels:

Total Cholesterol Level	Category
Less than 200 mg/dL	Desirable
200 - 239 mg/dL	Borderline high
240 mg/dL and above	High

LDL Cholesterol Level	Category
Less than 100 mg/dL	Optimal
100 - 129 mg/dL	Near optimal/above optimal
130 - 159 mg/dL	Borderline high
160 - 189 mg/dL	High
190 mg/dL and above	Very High

HDL Cholesterol Level	Category
60 mg/dL or above	Optimal
40 - 60 mg/dL	Near optimal
Less than 40 mg/dL	Too low

Triglyceride Level	Category
Less than 150 mg/dL	Normal
150 - 199 mg/dL	Borderline high
200 - 499 mg/dL	High
500 mg/dL and above	Very high

If you have:
1. lowered your total cholesterol
2. lowered your LDL cholesterol
3. lowered your triglycerides
4. raised your HDL cholesterol

Your potential rewards are a:
- significantly reduced chance of CHD
- lower chance of having a heart attack
- lower chance of needing bypass surgery or angioplasty
- lower chance of dying of CHD related conditions

FACTORS INFLUENCING YOUR BLOOD CHOLESTEROL LEVELS

Your blood cholesterol levels are influenced by a variety of factors.   Research has established that all of the following factors have some influence on your blood cholesterol levels to one degree or another.

- Heredity
- Foods you eat
- Physical activity
- Weight
- Stress
- Smoking
- Gender
- Age

Of the factors you can manage and control, the quantity and kinds of foods you eat have some of the greatest influence on your blood cholesterol level.

You can also manage and control your physical activity, weight, stress and smoking. However, you cannot change gender, age and heredity. So, do something about those circumstances you can manage and control to bring balance to those circumstances you cannot control.

Foods You Eat: The Difference Makes a Difference

Reducing the amount of saturated fat and cholesterol that you eat helps control your blood cholesterol level.

Some Facts to Remember:

- Saturated fat in the diet is the number one villain in causing blood cholesterol to go higher.
- Cholesterol in foods also contributes to raising blood cholesterol but to a much lesser degree than saturated fat.
- Polyunsaturated fat lowers blood cholesterol, but it lowers both the "bad" LDLs and the "good" HDLs.
- Monounsaturated fat lowers only the "bad" LDL cholesterol which is what you want. Canola and olive oils are the best sources of monounsaturated fats and should be used in place of other vegetable oils as much as possible.

Physical Activity: A Must for Everyone

Scientific research indicates that a sedentary lifestyle may significantly lower an individual's "good" HDLs and contribute to high blood cholesterol and overweight.

Moderate and regular physical activity tends to:

- Raise the "good" HDLs
- Lower triglycerides
- Lower LDLs
- Help you lose weight

Not being physically active is a risk factor for heart disease. You should try to be physically active for at least 30 minutes on most, if not all, days.

Weight: Something That May Need to Be Considered

Studies show that overweight individuals tend to have higher levels of blood cholesterol and of the "bad" LDLs than do those of recommended weight.

Being overweight is usually the result of an intake of calories (especially from highly starchy and highly sweet carbohydrates) that exceeds the needs of your body. These extra calories are converted into the fat triglyceride. It is believed that triglycerides are involved in the development of arteriosclerosis. So if you have never been motivated enough before to decrease the calories and/or the type of foods you eat, take heed, become motivated and increase the quality and length of your life.

Losing weight can help lower your triglyceride, LDL and total cholesterol levels as well as raise your HDL level.

Stress: Maybe Some Changes Are Needed

Stress may raise cholesterol levels, but it is possible that other factors may be the cause for the rise in blood cholesterol. For example, during periods of stress people may eat more foods that are high in saturated fat and cholesterol, and are highly starchy or highly sweet which may increase their cholesterol and triglyceride levels rather than the stress itself. This is a chicken and egg story, which came first?

Stress can be caused by how you are processing information rather than the information itself causing the stress. Human beings are able to manage short term periods of stress with no lasting effects. But when stress is prolonged it results in distress.

Smoking: Stop!

Cigarette smoking raises the risk of CHD. It lowers the "good" HDL cholesterol. The more cigarettes smoked, the lower the HDLs go. Smoking may also change LDL cholesterol to a form that promotes the buildup of deposits in the walls of the coronary arteries. If you are still smoking in this day and age after all the other dialogue against smoking, what can we say except, stop! Smoking leads to suffering and death for many while making money for many others.

Gender and Age: They Are What They Are

As women and men become older, their cholesterol levels rise. Women, before menopause, have lower total cholesterol levels than do men of the same age. After menopause, women's LDLs tend to increase.

Heredity: May Need to Be More Conscientious in Your Efforts to Control Your Cholesterol

You inherit tendencies toward certain blood cholesterol and blood triglyceride levels. One extreme example is the situation where approximately 1 in 500 individuals has a genetic problem of too few LDL receptors on his/her cells causing a high LDL cholesterol. If you have a high cholesterol level which will not come down even when doing all the "correct" things, for a long enough period of time, get checked for a genetic cause. If you have a genetic disorder contributing to a high cholesterol, then all of your blood relatives, including children over 2 and adolescents, should also have their cholesterol levels checked.

WHAT'S NEXT?

Now that you have a better understanding of your blood cholesterol, you should have a clearer reason for seeing the importance of taking an interest in your own personal well-being. See your physician and have your total lipid profile (total cholesterol, HDLs, VLDLS, LDLs, triglycerides) checked. For the method to follow, see the chapter, How To Determine If You Have A Cholesterol Problem.

2

HOW SERIOUS IS HIGH CHOLESTEROL?

There are important reasons for you to be concerned about the level of your cholesterol. High cholesterol increases the risk of atherosclerosis (ath-er-o-scle-ro-sis) which increases the risk of disorders of the cardiovascular (circulatory) system. The cardiovascular system consists of the heart and all the blood vessels (arteries, veins, and capillaries).

Atherosclerosis contributes directly to:

- Coronary Heart Disease (CHD)
- Stroke
- Other circulatory problems

In plain terms, high cholesterol can lead to atherosclerosis which can lead to a stroke, heart attack and/or other circulatory problems.

Your future and your overall well-being are directly related to how seriously you concern yourself with your own health care. You, yourself, are the only one who can do what is necessary to prevent cardiovascular disease. Don't take the risk of cardiovascular disease lightly; make certain that you and your doctor understand each other and work together for your well-being.

ATHEROSCLEROSIS

Atherosclerosis comes from the Greek word athero, meaning gruel or paste, and sclerosis, meaning hardness. Deposits of fatty substances, cholesterol, cellular waste, calcium and fibrin (clotting component in blood) build up in the inner lining of an artery. This buildup is called plaque. A partial or total blockage of blood flow through the artery may occur where there is plaque buildup. Atherosclerosis contributes directly to CHD and stroke.

Arteriosclerosis (ar-te-ri-o-scle-ro-sis) is a general term for the thickening and hardening of the arteries. Arteries are the blood vessels carrying blood, which contain oxygen and nutrients, from the heart to cells throughout the body. Normal healthy arteries have smooth muscular walls that propel the blood along toward the various body organs.

When the inner wall of an artery has rough plaque buildup, the artery narrows, the flow of blood slows, and a blood clot (thrombus) is more likely to form than in a healthy artery. The clot forms because blood is designed to clot when it comes in contact with foreign substances such as plaque.

Plaque buildup is a slow, progressive process that can begin even as early as childhood. In some people, the build up progresses rapidly in their thirties while in others it begins in their fifties or sixties. Most researchers of atherosclerosis believe this process begins because something damages the innermost layer of the artery and, over a period of time, substances from the bloodstream enter the artery wall. These substances gradually build up (plaque) and eventually narrow and block the artery.

The predominant fatty substance found in atherosclerotic plaque, is cholesterol.

Major potential causes of damage to the walls of your arteries include:

- Elevated levels of LDL cholesterol
- Low levels of HDL cholesterol
- Elevated levels of triglycerides
     especially in women and in diabetic patients
- Diabetes mellitus
- High blood pressure
- Cigarette smoking

Plaque may build up at various areas within your body but the most common areas appear to be:

- The carotid arteries, located in the neck which carry blood to the brain
- The coronary arteries, located in the heart muscle which carry blood to the heart itself
- The renal arteries carrying blood to the kidneys
- The femoral arteries carrying blood to the legs

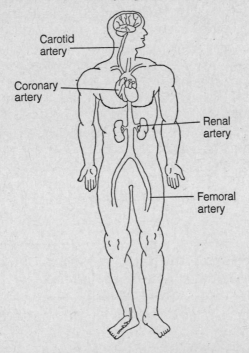

Coronary Heart Disease (CHD)

The human heart is a muscle which pumps blood throughout the body. The heart has its own blood vessels, the coronary arteries. Like any muscle, the heart needs a constant supply of oxygen and nutrients which are carried to it by the blood in the coronary arteries.

If the coronary arteries become clogged with fatty substances and cholesterol, they may become so narrow or completely blocked that the heart muscle no longer receives the quantity of oxygen and nutrients it needs. Chest pain (angina pectoris) may result. This may be the first symptom of heart disease. But some people never have angina and experience their first symptom as a heart attack which may be fatal.

The primary cause of heart attacks is coronary artery disease, which is caused by atherosclerosis.

There can be two results of coronary artery disease:

1. Heart muscle damage may result from a decreased flow of blood to an area of the heart because of partial blockage of the coronary arteries to that specific area.

2. Heart attack (myocardial infarction) results from a complete blockage of the blood flow to an area of the heart muscle (myocardium). That part of the heart muscle may actually die because it is deprived of the oxygen and nutrients its cells need. Depending on how much of the heart muscle is damaged, disability or death can result.

Regular exercise increases the collateral circulation in the heart muscle and helps deliver more blood to the heart muscle.

What is your risk of developing coronary heart disease or having a heart attack?

In general, the higher your LDL level and the more risk factors you have (other than LDL), the greater your chances of developing CHD or having a heart attack. Some people are at high risk for a heart attack because they already have CHD. Others are at high risk for developing CHD because they have diabetes (which is a strong risk factor) or a combination of risk factors for CHD.

A **risk factor** is a circumstance that increases your likelihood of getting a disease.

Follow the 3 steps below to discover your risk for developing CHD. If you find you have a high overall risk, then your goal will most likely be to lower your LDL cholesterol.

Step 1. Check the risk factors below to see how many you have

The following major risk factors that affect your LDL goal are:

- Cigarette smoking
- High blood pressure - 140/90 or higher or on blood pressure medication
- HDL cholesterol less than 40 mg/dL
- Family history of CHD
    CHD in father or brother before age 55
    CHD in mother or sister before age 65
- Age -   men 45 years or older
    women 55 years or older

Even though obesity and physical inactivity are not noted in the above list, they are conditions that need to be corrected.

Step 2. How many major risk factors do you have? If you have two or more, use the risk scoring tables on the following pages (which include your cholesterol levels) to find your risk score. Risk score refers to your chance of having a heart attack in the next ten years, given as a percentage.

(Use the Estimate of 10-Year Risk Charts; Framingham Point Scores on the following pages.)

My 10-year risk score is _____%.

Step 3. In the table below, use your medical history, number of risk factors, and risk score to find your risk of developing CHD or having a heart attack.

If You Have	You Are in Category
Heart disease, diabetes or risk score more than 20%*	I. Highest Risk
Two or more risk factors and risk score of 10 - 20 %	II. Next Highest Risk
Two or more risk factors and risk score less than 10 %	III. Moderate Risk
0 or 1 risk factor	IV. Low to Moderate Risk

My risk category is _____

* Means that more than 20 of 100 people in this category will have a heart attack within 10 years

Estimate of 10-Year risk for Men: NIH, National Heart, Lung and Blood Institute
(Framingham Point Scores)

Age	Points
20 - 34	-9
35 - 39	-4
40 - 44	0
45 - 49	3
50 - 54	6
55 - 59	8
60 - 64	10
65 - 69	11
70 - 74	12
75 - 79	13

HDL (mg/dL)	Points
≥ 60	- 1
50 - 59	0
40 - 49	1
< 40	2

Total Cholesterol	Points				
	Age 20-39	Age 40-49	Age 50-59	Age 60-69	Age 70-79
< 160	0	0	0	0	0
160 - 199	4	3	2	1	0
200 - 239	7	5	3	1	0
240 - 279	9	6	4	2	1
≥ 280	11	8	5	3	1

	Points				
Nonsmoker	0	0	0	0	0
Smoker	8	5	3	1	1

Systolic BP (mmHg)	If Untreated	If Treated
< 120	0	0
120 - 129	0	1
130 - 139	1	2
140 - 159	1	2
≥ 160	2	3

Point Total	10 - Year Risk %
< 0	< 1
0	1
1	1
2	1
3	1
4	1
5	2
6	2
7	3
8	4
9	5
10	6
11	8
12	10
13	12
14	16
15	20
16	25
≥ 17	≥ 30

10 - Year risk _____%

Estimate of 10-Year Risk for Women: (Framingham Point Scores)

NIH, National Heart, Lung and Blood Institute

Age	Points
20 - 34	-7
35 - 39	-3
40 - 44	0
45 - 49	3
50 - 54	6
55 - 59	8
60 - 64	10
65 - 69	12
70 - 74	14
75 - 79	16

HDL (mg/dL)	Points
≥ 60	-1
50 - 59	0
40 - 49	1
< 40	2

Total Cholesterol	Points				
	Age 20-39	Age 40-49	Age 50-59	Age 60-69	Age 70-79
< 160	0	0	0	0	0
160 - 199	4	3	2	1	1
200 - 239	8	6	4	2	1
240 - 279	11	8	5	3	2
≥ 280	13	10	7	4	2

	Points				
Nonsmoker	0	0	0	0	0
Smoker	9	7	4	2	1

Systolic BP (mmHg)	If Untreated	If Treated
< 120	0	0
120 - 129	1	3
130 - 139	2	4
140 - 159	3	5
≥ 160	4	6

Point Total	10 - Year Risk %
< 9	< 1
9	1
10	1
11	1
12	1
13	2
14	2
15	3
16	4
17	5
18	6
19	8
20	11
21	17
22	17
23	22
24	27
≥ 25	≥ 30

10 - Year risk _____ %

Three risk categories that modify LDL cholesterol goals

Your physician will take your risk factors into account in determining your LDL cholesterol goal (level).

Risk Category	LDL Goal
1. If you have CHD or CHD risk equivalents*	less than 100
2. If you have 2 or more risk factors	less than 130
3. If you have zero to one risk factor	less than 160

*CHD risk equivalents are:

- Other clinical forms of arteriosclerosis disease (peripheral arterial disease, abdominal aortic aneurysm and symptomatic carotid artery disease).

- Diabetes

- Multiple risk factors that confer a 10 year risk for heart disease > 20 %

Attention!!!
Your children over 2 years of age should be tested if there is a biological family history of:

- **parent, sibling, grandparent, aunt or uncle who experienced one of the following before age 55:**

  - **angina pectoris (chest pain)**
  - **heart attack**
  - **peripheral vascular disease**
  - **stroke**
  - **sudden cardiac death**
  - **coronary atherosclerosis**

Special Concerns

People with LDL cholesterol 190 or over usually have a genetic form of hypercholesterolemia. Early detection of this through cholesterol testing in young adults is needed to prevent premature coronary heart disease. Family testing is important to identify similarly affected relatives. This disorder often requires combined drug therapy to achieve the goals of LDL-lowering therapy.

In rare instances some individuals have triglycerides of 500 or more. The initial aim of therapy is to prevent acute pancreatitis by lowering their triglycerides. To do this requires a very low fat diet with only 15% or less of the total calories coming from fat along with weight reduction, increased physical activity and usually a triglyceride-lowering medication.

Metabolic Syndrome

The risk for CHD is influenced by other factors not included among the major risk factors.

Many people have a group of risk factors that make up a condition called the "metabolic syndrome". Components characteristic of the metabolic syndrome are:

- abdominal obesity
- elevated triglycerides
- low HDL cholesterol
- elevated blood pressure
- insulin resistance - the normal actions of insulin are impaired. This is promoted by obesity (particularly abdominal obesity) and physical inactivity. But some people are genetically predisposed to insulin resistance.

Evidence is accumulating that the risk for CHD can be reduced by modification of the above risk factors.

A combination of the above risk factors increase the risk for CHD at any given LDL cholesterol level. The diagnosis of metabolic syndrome is made when three or more of the risk factors below are present.

Risk Factors	Defining Level
Abdominal Obesity* Men women	Waist Circumference† >40" (> 102cm) >35" (> 88cm)
Triglycerides	≥ 150 mg/dL
HDL Cholesterol Men Women	 <40 mg/dL <50 mg/dL
Blood pressure	≥130/≥85
Fasting blood glucose	≥110 mg/dL

Key: > more than   < less than

* Overweight and obesity are associated with insulin resistance and the metabolic syndrome. However, the presence of abdominal obesity is more correlated with the metabolic risk factors than is an elevated body mass index (BMI). Therefore, the simple measure of waist circumstance is recommended to identity the body weight component of the metabolic syndrome.

† Some men can develop multiple metabolic risk factors when the waist circumstance is only marginally increased, e.g. 37-39" (94-102 cm). Such men may have a strong genetic contribution to insulin resistance. They should benefit from changes in life habits, similarly to men with categorical increases in waist circumstance.

The first-line of therapies for all risk factors associated with metabolic syndrome are:

• weight reduction
• increased physical activity

Therefore, if metabolic syndrome is present after appropriate control of LDL cholesterol then weight reduction and physical activity should be emphasized.

CHD is the number one cause of death of men and women in America. Statistics indicate that approximately 1,250,000 people suffer from a heart attack annually. About 500,000 people die from heart disease annually.

Even though heart attacks are the number one cause of death in America, you can greatly help protect yourself and your loved ones by slight changes in:

• What you eat
• Your lifestyle

Heart attack warning signs

• Uncomfortable pressure, fullness, squeezing or pain in the center of the chest that lasts more than a few minutes, or goes away and comes back

• Pain that spreads to the shoulders, neck or arms

• Chest discomfort with lightheadedness, fainting, sweating, nausea or shortness of breath

Not all of these warning signs occur in every heart attack. If some start to occur, **DON'T WAIT.** Get help immediately, don't drive yourself to your doctor or emergency room! **Call 911.**

Stroke

Stroke is one form of cardiovascular disease. It is an injury to the nervous system which occurs when an adequate supply of blood carrying oxygen and nutrients is prevented from reaching portions of the brain. The inadequate supply of oxygen and nutrients is often the result of an obstruction of the flow of blood in or to the brain. Causes of obstruction are a clot or a buildup of plaque in an artery leading to or in the brain.

Most often a clot forms in the artery at the site of the blockage. But some times a clot breaks off from an artery somewhere else in the body and travels through the larger blood vessels until it becomes wedged in a smaller cerebral (brain) artery. Brain cells quickly deteriorate and die when they are deprived of the oxygen rich blood normally supplied by the artery.

When the cells die, that area of the brain no longer functions. Subsequently, the part of the body controlled by this area of the brain can't function, causing unconsciousness, paralysis of part of the body, and impairment of speech, vision, thought and memory patterns. All of these effects may range from mild to severe, and from treatable to permanent. The severity of the problem depends on the extent and location of brain cell damage and the ability of the body to compensate and restore a blood supply to injured areas of the brain.

Recent research indicates that high triglycerides and low HDLs in people with CHD are risk factors for having a stroke.

A stroke is usually the culmination of a progressive disease that may extend over many years and is not always detectable in a routine physical examination. One helpful exam is the doctor listening to the blood flow through the carotid arteries in your neck. These arteries carry the blood to your brain.

Since in many cases there are no warning signs, a stroke is a particularly terrifying event. Approximately 500,000 Americans suffer a stroke each year. A stroke may not be fatal but can be a major cause of disability.

Stroke warning signs

- Sudden numbness or weakness of the face, arm or leg, especially on one side of the body

- Sudden confusion, trouble speaking or understanding

- Sudden trouble seeing in one or both eyes

- Sudden trouble walking, dizziness, loss of balance or coordination

- Sudden, severe headache with no known cause

Not all of these warning signs occur in every stroke. If some start to occur, **DON'T WAIT.** Get help immediately, don't drive yourself to your doctor or emergency room! **Call 911**

Your number one protection against having a stroke is the food and behavior modification plan presented in this book! Consider using the information immediately!

Other Circulatory Problems

Just as the arteries supplying blood to the brain and heart may have atherosclerosis so can the arteries supplying other areas of the body. For example this can occur in the renal arteries leading to the kidneys and the femoral arteries leading to the lower part of the legs.

If blockage occurs in the femoral artery, a condition known as arteriosclerosis obliterans may occur. This condition is most common in men over the age of 50 who:

• Smoke
• Have high cholesterol
• May also have diabetes

Depending on where the artery in the leg is blocked, the location of the pain resulting from the blockage can range from the hip to the foot. Ulcers on the foot, toes and/or heel may develop due to the lack of sufficient oxygen and nutrients being supplied to the area. The most severe result would be gangrene of the affected area and possible amputation of the affected limb.

If you haven't understood it before, understand it now: a change in lifestyle (stop smoking; exercise more, etc.) and the foods you eat are of primary importance for avoidance of circulatory problems.

3

HOW TO DETERMINE IF YOU HAVE A CHOLESTEROL PROBLEM

Most often with your health, you are concerned with how well you feel and look, and you leave it at that. However, with the concern of cholesterol, it is not a matter of how well you feel or look but how well your cardiovascular system (heart and blood vessels) is functioning. Unlike most health conditions, there are no telltale symptoms to warn you if your cholesterol is high.

The cardiovascular conditions that high cholesterol can lead to cause symptoms only after the damage has been done. Therefore, it is your responsibility to find out what your cholesterol level is before you have any cardiovascular symptoms and hopefully avoid ever having any problems. Sounds like a pure and simple case for preventive medicine.

In choosing a physician, be certain he/she can communicate easily and is knowledgeable about cholesterol/CHD, and does not just use a few "buzz words." You should feel comfortable asking questions and feel that the questions are answered with a true interest, concern and knowledge. In some respects, choosing the right physician to help you is the most important thing you can do.

GET THE TEST: THE TOTAL LIPID PROFILE

Every adult age twenty and over should be tested every five years. If there is a family history (parents, grandparents, aunts and uncles) of high cholesterol and/or coronary heart disease before age 55, a child should be tested soon after the age of two. If the results are within the normal range, the test should be repeated every five years. Be certain to keep a running record of the test results in a safe place so you can see if there is any great change occurring over the years. See chapter, Cholesterol Concerns of Children and Adolescents.

Take special note; there are two different tests for determining your cholesterol level:

1. TOTAL CHOLESTEROL TEST
2. TOTAL LIPID PROFILE (Lipoprotein Analysis) which includes the following components:

   1) Total cholesterol
   2) LDL cholesterol
   3) HDL cholesterol
   4) Triglycerides
   5) VLDL cholesterol - not always included

For your first test, possibly only the total cholesterol will be ordered. This is not the better way to go because it's possible for your total cholesterol to be within the "desirable" range, but for one of the components (LDLs, HDLs, triglycerides) to be too high or too low. If you or your doctor were not aware of these high or low values, then you would not be treated according to your real needs and your risk of having a medical problem would not be discovered and resolved. You would have a false sense of security because you wouldn't know all of the information necessary for a complete picture. Get the complete picture by getting complete information. This can only be accomplished by having the complete test. Get the TOTAL LIPID PROFILE TEST!

The best procedure for determining your cholesterol level:

- Ask your doctor to order a total lipid profile test (total cholesterol, HDLs, LDLs, VLDLs, triglycerides).

- Fast nine to twelve hours before the test to permit a more accurate test of the triglyceride level which rises appreciably after eating. Avoid alcohol for 24 hours before the test. In general, the most favorable time to have the test is between 7 and 9 am after having not eaten from 9 pm the night before. Only water is permitted during this time.

- Sit for at least 5 minutes before your blood is drawn. Sit (do not lie down or stand) when your blood is being drawn. The tourniquet should be used for as brief a time as possible, less than a minute.

It is most important that you get this test immediately!

NOTE:
- Do not have the test taken:
    - Just after you have been seriously ill
    - Within three months of a heart attack
    - During the last trimester of pregnancy
    - After a major weight loss
    - After sudden dietary changes
    These situations interfere with a true cholesterol reading.

- Since there have been labs which have not performed the test according to professional standards, call the lab where you plan to have the blood sample taken and ask if:
    - It is accredited by a national agency, such as the College of American Pathology.
    - Its equipment is checked daily.
    - Its testing results are audited regularly by an independent agency.
    You want to have the test performed in a lab that answers yes to these questions. In addition you may ask to see their certificate of accreditation.
- Always have your test performed at the same lab.

CHOLESTEROL NUMBERS GAME, UNDERSTANDING IT

Blood cholesterol is measured in milligrams per deciliter; a deciliter is approximately one-tenth of a quart. If your cholesterol is 189 mg/dl, this means that the cholesterol found in a deciliter of liquid weighs 189 milligrams. For comparison, 28,350 milligrams equals only 1 ounce.

In order to determine whether you have high cholesterol, the values (numbers) of all of your blood lipids (cholesterol, HDLs, LDLs, triglycerides) need to be known. These values and other risk factors are used to indicate your risk of developing cardiovascular disease. A few days after you have had your cholesterol test, your doctor will receive the test results and should give you specific information as to what these numbers mean.

It is most important that you do not content yourself with a general statement that the test was "normal" or "okay"; get the specific numbers. Ask questions and talk them out with your doctor. Your doctor is your foremost health adviser and is the best source for the scientific information required to understand your body chemistry.

Ask for and get a copy of the test results for your records; compare them with the charts below and keep them in a safe place so they can be compared with your future tests results over the years.

Classification of Cholesterol Levels For Adults

Total Cholesterol Level	Category
Less than 200 mg/dL	Desirable
200 - 239 mg/dL	Borderline high
240 mg/dL and above	High

LDL Cholesterol Level	Category
Less than 100 mg/dL	Optimal
100 - 129 mg/dL	Near optimal/above optimal
130 - 159 mg/dL	Borderline high
160 - 189 mg/dL	High
190 mg/dL and above	Very High

HDL Cholesterol Level

HDL Cholesterol Level	Category
60 mg/dL or above	Optimal
40 - 60 mg/dL	Near optimal
Less than 40 mg/dL	Too low

Triglyceride Level

Triglyceride Level	Category
Less than 150 mg/dL	Normal
150 - 199 mg/dL	Borderline high
200 - 499 mg/dL	High
500 mg/dL and above	Very high

Source: National Heart, Lung, and Blood Institute

Attention!!!
Your children over 2 years of age should be tested if either of the biological parents has or ever had a high cholesterol (above 240).

VISUAL AIDS TO HELP TRACK YOUR PROGRESS

It is a good idea to keep a running record of your cholesterol test results so you can see the progress you are making. Enter in the chart below your test results as soon as you receive them so you will have the benefit of a on going record.

PERSONAL CHOLESTEROL RECORD				
	Initial test	6 Weeks test	3$^1/_2$ Months test	6$^1/_2$ Months test
Cholesterol				
LDLs				
HDLs				
Triglycerides				

Using your test result numbers, you can make right angle graphs to plot your progress of lowering your Total Cholesterol, LDLs, Triglycerides, and raising your HDLs. The graphs enable you to visualize your progress. We have shown a model graph with a blank one along side for your own personal use.

SAMPLE GRAPHS

Total Cholesterol Chart

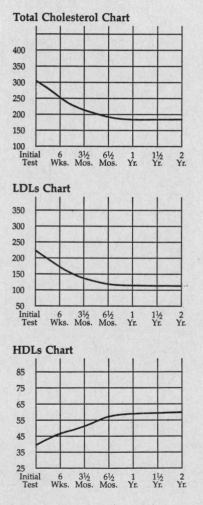

Your Total Cholesterol Chart

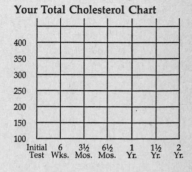

LDLs Chart

Your LDLs Chart

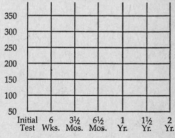

HDLs Chart

Your HDLs Chart

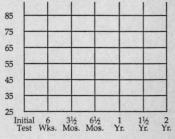

Triglyceride Chart

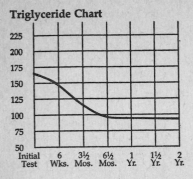

Your Triglyceride Chart

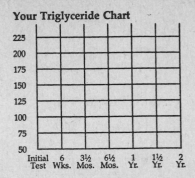

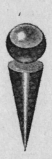

4

HOW TO CONTROL YOUR CHOLESTEROL

This chapter explains the basic facts about controlling your blood cholesterol. If you wish to learn more about cholesterol, just read the additional chapters where we give information in greater detail. The more you read the more you will learn about blood cholesterol and your body chemistry and the more clearly you will understand how they fit together.

The main goal of cholesterol control treatment is to lower your LDL level enough to reduce your risk of developing coronary heart disease (CHD) or having a heart attack or stroke. The higher your risk, the lower your LDL goal will be. To find your LDL goal, see chapter two.

By closely following the correct plan and monitoring your progress with regular medical checkups, you can control your blood cholesterol levels and greatly reduce your risk of developing a cardiovascular disease. Generally, both your total cholesterol and LDL levels will begin to drop within 1 to 3 weeks after you begin your cholesterol controlling program.

> **Lower total cholesterol, LDLs and triglycerides and higher HDLs results in a happy heart because of a lower risk of coronary heart disease and stroke.**

How rapidly you lower your cholesterol levels and how low it falls depend on a few key factors:

- *The amount of saturated fat in your diet before beginning the program.* If you have been eating high amounts of saturated fats rather than moderate to low amounts, you will probably see a greater reduction in your cholesterol level when you start to change your eating style.

- *Your cholesterol level before starting the program.* In general, the higher your cholesterol level, the greater percentage of reduction you can expect.

- *How responsive your body is to your new diet.* Genetic factors play a role in determining your cholesterol level and to some extent, can determine your body's responsiveness to the cholesterol lowering program.

- *How thoroughly you follow the cholesterol lowering program.* Are you eating significantly less fat and cholesterol? Are you eating more high soluble fiber foods? Are you being physically active regularly?

Because there are so many variables, such as age, gender, heredity, etc., some individuals will make more progress than others.

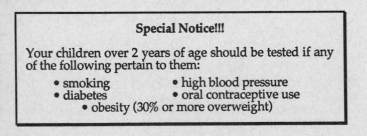

Special Notice!!!

Your children over 2 years of age should be tested if any of the following pertain to them:
- smoking
- diabetes
- high blood pressure
- oral contraceptive use
- obesity (30% or more overweight)

THE NATIONAL CHOLESTEROL EDUCATION PROGRAM FOR LOWERING YOUR CHOLESTEROL

Nothing works better than the way it is organized and managed. The easiest way to be successful in any project is to organize it in a way that allows you to follow through and manage it in the most beneficial manner. With this in mind, we have tried to present the following information in an organized way so that it can be easily understood and managed to achieve the best and quickest results. We have tried our best. The rest of the job is up to you.

Two Main Ways to Control Your Cholesterol

1. Therapeutic Lifestyle Changes (TLC) - for those whose LDL is above goal level. The TLC is comprised of:

   A. Cholesterol lowering diet (TLC Diet)

   B. Increase physical activity

   C. Weight management

2. Medications - if cholesterol lowering medications are needed, they are used together with TLC to help lower your LDL cholesterol level.

Whether your cholesterol is high because of heredity, diet or a combination of both, your doctor will prescribe a change in the foods you eat as the first thing for lowering your cholesterol. Eating correctly day by day is essential for lowering your cholesterol as many scientific studies have shown. The second most important thing you should do is regular, moderate physical activity. By following the above, you will usually lose weight if necessary.

Below are the various risk categories with their LDL goal and what you should do to attain your LDL goal in relation to your risk. To determine your category, see What is Your Risk of Developing Coronary Heart Disease Or Having a Heart Attack in Chapter 2.

What To Do For Your Risk Category

If your category is:

Category I, Highest Risk, your LDL goal is less than 100.

- If your LDL is below 100:
  You should follow the TLC diet on your own to keep your LDL as low as possible.

- If your LDL is 100 or above:
  You will need to begin the TLC.

- If your LDL is 100 to 129:
  You may need to consider medication along with the TLC.

- If your LDL is 130 or higher
  You may need to begin medication along with the TLC.

Category II, Next Highest Risk, your LDL goal is less than 130.

- If your LDL is less than 130:
  You will need to follow the Heart-Healthy diet*.

- If your LDL is 130 or above:
  You will need the begin the TLC.

- If you LDL is 130 or above after 3 months of the TLC:
  You may need medication along with the TLC.

Category III, Moderate Risk, your LDL goal is less than 130.

- If your LDL is less than 130:
  You will need to follow the Heart-healthy diet*.

- If your LDL is 130 or above:
  You will to begin the TLC.

- If your LDL is 160 or above after 3 months of the TLC:
  You may need medication along with the TLC.

<u>Category IV,</u> **Low to Moderate Risk,** your LDL goal is less than 160.

- If your LDL is less than 160:
  You will need to follow the Heart-healthy diet*.

- If you LDL is 160 or above:
  You will need to begin the TLC.

- If your LDL is 160 or above after 3 months of the TLC:

  You may need medication along with the TLC, especially if your LDL is 190 or above.

---

* Heart- healthy diet:
  Total fat: 30% or less of total daily calories
  Saturated fat: 8-10% of total daily calories
  Cholesterol: less than 300 mg daily
  Sodium: up to 240 mg daily
  Calories: just enough to achieve or maintain a healthy weight
    and reduce cholesterol level if necessary

Source: National Institutes of Health

THERAPEUTIC LIFESTYLE CHANGES (TLC)

A. Cholesterol Lowering Diet (TLC diet)

The changes in the foods you eat will be subtle and appear to be small, but the difference in your body chemistry will be dramatic and significant. If you never have agreed with or understood the statement, "You become what you have eaten", understand it now as a perfect representation of how your body chemistry reflects what you have eaten. Dietary changes are very important for lowering and controlling your cholesterol levels.

Four features of the diet:

1. Reduce intake of fat, especially saturated fat
2. Reduce intake of cholesterol

3. Eat more complex carbohydrates, especially those containing soluble fiber (10-25 g/day)
4. Consider the use of plant stanols/sterols found in products such as Benacol and Take Control (vegetable oil spreads)

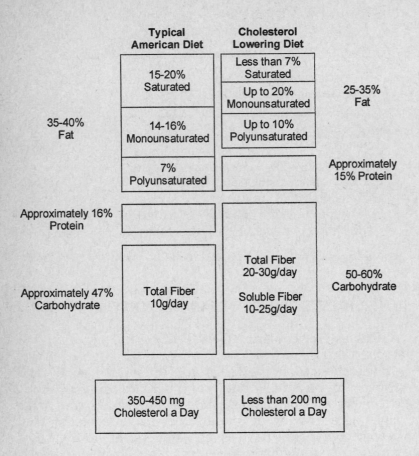

To enable you to know the specific fat, cholesterol and carbohydrate content of commonly eaten foods, you need to read labels and buy a book containing this information. See book information in the back of this book.

1. Reduce intake of fat, especially saturated fat

The typical American gets about 35% to 40% of his/her total calories from fat. The National Cholesterol Education program strongly recommends that you should get no more than 25% to 35% of your total daily calories from fat.

Reasons for eating less fat:

* To make it easier to reduce saturated fat intake which will help decrease your cholesterol level
* To promote weight reduction in overweight individuals by substituting foods with less calories. Remember, one gram of fat has 9 calories while one gram of protein or carbohydrate has only 4 calories.

There are two major categories of dietary fat:

1. Saturated fat
2. Unsaturated fat--comprised of two types of fat:
   polyunsaturated fat   (poly-un-sat-u-rated)
   monounsaturated fat   (mono-un-sat-u-rated)

All foods containing fat are comprised of a mixture of the above fats. The combination of these fats in the foods you eat make up the total amount of fat you eat daily. Following is the recommended percentage of daily total calories you may have from each type of fat:

1. Saturated fat.. less than 7 %
2. Unsaturated fat
   polyunsaturated fat... up to 10 %
   monounsaturated fat....................................... up to 20 %

Saturated Fat

The most effective way to lower your cholesterol is to eat less saturated fat. It is very important that less than 7% of your total daily calories come from saturated fat because research has established; **it is saturated fat that raises blood cholesterol more than anything else you eat, even more than the cholesterol you eat.**

The major sources of saturated fats are:
- Animal products (meats, whole milk and its products)
- Hydrogenated vegetable oils = trans fatty acids which appear to raise cholesterol more than unsaturated fats; found mostly in margarines and commercially baked items.
- Three vegetable oils (coconut oil, palm and palm kernel oils, and cocoa butter)

Saturated fats are solid at room temperature whereas unsaturated fats are liquid at room temperature.

Foods to avoid in order to eat less saturated fats

The most common foods to avoid are:
- Fat on a cut of meat
- Sausage and processed luncheon meats
- Skin of poultry
- Butter
- Whole milk cheese
- Whole milk, 2% milk and cream
- Ice cream
- Solid vegetable shortenings
- Hydrogenated vegetable oils - found frequently in margarines and commercially baked items
- Lard
- Commercially baked goods containing one or more of the following:
     Coconut oil
     Cocoa butter--found in chocolate
     Palm kernel oil
     Palm oil
- Nondairy coffee creamers -- usually contain palm or
  . coconut oil
- Hot chocolate mixes--usually contain palm or coconut oil
- Prepared breakfast drinks--may contain palm or coconut oil

Because most fats are not able to be seen in products, you must carefully read the labels on packaged foods to determine what the fat content is. Many labels list what oils and/or shortenings are in the product, and some may list how much saturated fat there is per serving. Using this information will help you decide which foods are appropriate for you. For more label information, see Reading and Understanding Labels in the chapter, Food Logistics.

Foods to use to replace high saturated fat foods

Try using low fat products such as:

- Lean cuts of meat: trim all visible fat--bake, roast or broil rather than fry

- Fish and white meat of poultry--have less saturated fat than red or dark meat

- Whole grains and legumes in place of red meat

- Tofu, a soybean product, in place of red meat

- Soft or liquid (not hard) margarine--read labels and use the one with the least amount of saturated fat and an acceptable liquid vegetable oil listed first

- Low fat cheeses--part skim mozzarella, part skim ricotta, 1% cottage, sapsago (high in sodium)

- Low fat or nonfat yogurt in place of sour cream (add chives)

- Low fat (1%) or skim milk

- Ice milk, light ice cream or sherbet--for special occasions only

- Sorbet

- Home made baked goods made with canola or olive oil

> In general, food products from land animals contain saturated fat, whereas those from water animals contain unsaturated fat.

Unsaturated Fat

Of your total caloric intake, up to 30% of your calories may come from unsaturated fats. These fats are liquid at room temperature and are found primarily in vegetable oils (except cocoa butter, coconut, palm and palm kernel oils) and fish oils. Current research shows that the unsaturated omega-3 fatty acids which are found in fish have been linked with lower rates of heart attacks. It is suggested that you have fish two to three times a week in place of red meat and poultry.

Remember, there are two types of unsaturated fats:

1. Polyunsaturated
2. Monounsaturated

Polyunsaturated fats may comprise up to 10% of your total caloric intake. They help to lower your cholesterol by lowering both the "bad" LDL cholesterol and the "good" HDL cholesterol. However, you do not want your HDLs lowered but left the same or raised. Therefore, although you do need some polyunsaturated fats in your diet, you don't want to over use them.

Polyunsaturated fats are found primarily in:

- Corn oil
- Cottonseed oil
- Safflower oil
- Sesame oil
- Soybean oil
- Sunflower oil
- Walnut oil
- Wheat germ oil

Monounsaturated fats may comprise up to 20% of your total daily caloric intake. They lower only the "bad" LDL cholesterol, which is what you want, while the "good" HDLs stay about the same. This is beneficial in relation to your overall cholesterol situation.

It has been observed that in Mediterranean countries such as Greece, Crete and southern Italy there is a low rate of heart disease and low cholesterol levels even though the people have diets high in olive oil. In fact, studies in the United States have shown that those who ate more mono-unsaturated fats had lower levels of "bad" LDLs than those who ate just a low fat diet.

The best sources of monounsaturated fats are:

- Avocado oil
- Canola oil, made from rapeseed
- Olive oil

When cooking and baking it is preferable to use vege-table oils high in monounsaturated fats and low in sat-urated fat such as canola oil and olive oil.

How to Determine the Amount of Fat You May Eat Daily

It may seem somewhat of an overkill to belabor the aspect of determining the amounts of the different types of fat permitted; we agree. In most cases you don't have to do all this nit-picking and calculating if you simply stop eating the saturated fat foods, such as butter, whole milk products, poultry skin, fatty meats and bakery goods made with palm, palm kernel and/or coconut oils. But, if you are one who requires and/or desires more information, by all means make the effort.

It's important to note that fat contains more than twice the amount of calories per gram weight as protein or carbohydrate. A gram of fat has 9 calories and a gram of protein or carbohydrate has only 4 calories.

There are two steps for determining the amount of fat (hidden and visible) you may eat per day:

1. Decide how many total calories you should have per day. The chart below is an overall average of caloric intake for various ages and weights.

RECOMMENDED DAILY CALORIE ALLOWANCE			
Age	Wt.	Ht.	Calories
Males 19-22	147lb.	69	3000
23-50	154	69	2700
51+	154	69	2400
Females 19-22	128 lb.	65	2100
23-50	128	65	2000
51+	128	65	1800

Source: Food and Nutrition Board, National Academy of Science/National Research Council

2. Once you have decided how many calories you desire or need per day from the above chart, look at the chart below to determine how many grams of fat you are permitted daily. Remember, you are to get only 25% to 35% of your daily calories from the fat you eat.

Remember, if you decrease the amount of calories you are getting from fat, you may want to replace those calories by eating more complex carbohydrates. Of course this is based on the criteria of your individual situation of whether or not you need to lose weight.

Permissible Amount of Fat to Provide 25%, 30%, or 35% of Daily Calories at Specific Calorie Levels			
Calories per day	Grams of total fat that provide		
	25% of calories	30% of calories	35% of calories
	Grams	Grams	Grams
1500	42	50	58
1800	50	60	70
2000	56	66	78
2100	58	70	82
2400	67	80	93
2700	75	90	105
2800	78	93	109
3000	83	100	117

If you desire, you can determine how many grams of each type of fat you may eat daily based on the percentage of each fat allowed.

Saturated fat........................ less than 7% of total daily calories
Polyunsaturated fat................ up to 10% of total daily calories
Monounsaturated fat .... up to 20% of total daily calories

Calculate your grams of each type of fat by multiplying the percentage times your total daily calories and then divide that answer by 9 (the number of calories in a gram of fat). The resulting number is the grams of that type of fat you are permitted daily.

For example: If you decide to eat a total of 1800 calories a day with 30% of the calories being fat, multiple 1800 by the percentage of each type of fat (the total percentage of the three fats should be 30%), then divide by 9.

Saturated fat = 5% of total calories (1800) = .05 x 1800 = 90 calories divided by 9 (calories per gram) = 10 grams per day.

Polyunsaturated fat = 10% of total calories = .10 x 1800 = 180 calories divided by 9 = 20 grams per day.

Monounsaturated fat = 15% of total calories = .15 x 1800 = 270 calories divided by 9 = 30 grams per day.

Thus you may eat:

Saturated fat	10 grams
Polyunsaturated fat	20 grams
Monounsaturated fat	30 grams
a total of	60 grams of fat daily

Most food labels will list the total amount of fat per serving. Some will also list saturated fat, polyunsaturated fat and monounsaturated fat. If only two of the specific fats are listed, you can subtract them from the total fat to discover how much there is of the third fat.

You may want to avoid products that do not list the types and amounts of various fats. See the section Reading and Understanding Labels in the chapter on Food Logistics.

Hydrogenated and Partially Hydrogenated Oils

One last word about fats. You will see the words hydrogenated and partially hydrogenated on ingredients list. These terms mean that unsaturated vegetable oils have undergone a process to make them more saturated, subsequently solid. These hydrogenated oils are used in various products such as solid vegetable shortenings, margarines and commercially baked goods to prolong their shelf life. These oils should be avoided. They are referred to as trans-fatty acids and gram for gram can increase bad LDL cholesterol almost as much as saturated fat.

2. Reduce intake of cholesterol

You would think that if your blood cholesterol is high, the most important thing you could do to lower it would be to stop eating all foods containing cholesterol. Ironically that's not true! Eating smaller quantities of foods containing cholesterol and foods lower in cholesterol content are the key points you want to remember.

Research tells us that the saturated fat you eat increases your blood cholesterol level more than the cholesterol you eat. You should however, still decrease the amount of cholesterol you usually eat.

The recommended daily intake of cholesterol is less than 200 mg., which is a little less than the amount of cholesterol in one egg yolk. The average American eats approximately 350 to 450 mg. of cholesterol a day. Easy math suggests the average American should cut back 150 mg. to 250 mg. of cholesterol a day.

Cholesterol is found only in foods of animal origin:

- Meats, poultry, fish and shellfish
- Milk and milk products
- Egg yolks

All meats and poultry contain about the same amount of cholesterol per ounce. Most fish and shellfish contain slightly less cholesterol per ounce, except shrimp which contains slightly more cholesterol than meats. Cholesterol is in the muscle and fat of these foods. Most of the cholesterol in milk is in the fat.

Cholesterol Content Of Some Common Foods:

Egg yolk	215 mg
1 cup whole milk	33 mg
1 cup skim (no milk solids added)	4 mg
3 oz. regular ground beef, cooked	76 mg
3 oz. sirloin steak, lean & fat, cooked	77 mg
3 oz. liver, fried	410 mg
3 oz. sweetbreads	400 mg
3 oz. veal cutlet, broiled	109 mg
3 oz. pork chop, broiled	79 mg
3 oz. lamb chop, braised	78 mg
3 oz. chicken breast with skin, cooked	73 mg
3 oz. chicken drum stick with skin, cooked	78 mg
3 oz. flounder without added fat, cooked	55 mg
3 oz. shellfish, cooked:	
Clams	57 mg
Crab meat	
Alaskan King	45 mg
Blue crab	85 mg
Lobster	61 mg
Oysters	93 mg
Scallops	35 mg
Shrimp	166 mg
1" cube cheddar cheese	18 mg
1 cup ice cream, vanilla (11% fat)	59 mg
1 cup frozen custard, soft serve	153 mg

1 cup sherbet (2% fat)	14 mg
1 cup frozen yogurt	13 mg
1 cup yogurt:	
made with whole milk	29 mg
made with lowfat milk	11 mg
made with nonfat milk	4 mg
1 slice cheesecake, $1/12$ of 9" cake	170 mg
1 slice angel food cake, any size	0 mg

The foods highest in cholesterol and which should be significantly limited are:

- Egg yolks
- Organ meats--liver, kidney, brain, sweetbreads, heart
- Full fat dairy products

For each whole egg called for in a recipe, you can usually substitute two egg whites.

Shellfish are not high in cholesterol as is commonly thought. Shrimp has the highest level--over 150 mg. per 3 oz. serving. You can work shrimp into your menu once in a while without any real problem. Scallops have a low 35 mg. per 3 oz. serving. Compare that figure with a 3 oz. serving of white meat of chicken at 54 mg. What you have to relate to when eating shellfish is how it has been prepared. Has it been fried? Was butter or another highly saturated fat used in the preparation?

Remember, there is no cholesterol in:

fruits	grains
vegetables	nuts
legumes	seeds

Read labels on packaged foods for cholesterol content per serving. However remember, when reading the listing of ingredients it is more important to be concerned with saturated fat than cholesterol. Beware of products whose labels state in large print on the front of the package, "NO CHOLESTEROL". They may still be high in saturated fat, which raises your blood cholesterol more severely than cholesterol itself. Look for a package whose label states "NO SATURATED FAT AND NO CHOLESTEROL."

3. Eat more complex carbohydrates, especially those containing soluble fiber

Carbohydrates should make up 50% to 60% of your total daily calories. Carbohydrates have no cholesterol, very little saturated fat, and some unsaturated fat. They come from plants and are the chief source of energy for all body functions and muscular exertion.

There are two categories of carbohydrates:

1. Simple carbohydrates--sugars found in and derived from fruits and vegetables.

2. Complex carbohydrates--starches and fiber found in vegetables, whole grains, legumes, nut, seeds and fruit.

When choosing whole grains - choose foods that name one of the following ingredients **first** on the label's ingredient list:

brown rice	popcorn	pearl barley
graham flour	oatmeal	whole grain corn
whole oats	whole rye	bulgur (cracked wheat)
whole wheat		

Try some of these whole grain foods:

whole wheat bread	whole wheat or whole rye crackers
oatmeal	whole grain ready-to-eat-cereal
tabouli salad	pearl barley or rice in soup
whole wheat pasta	

Note: "Wheat flour", "enriched flour" and "degerminated cornmeal" are not whole grains.

In nature, both the simple and complex carbohydrates come packaged together in fruits, vegetables, legumes, grains, nuts and seeds. Fruits have a greater concentration of simple carbohydrates than vegetables, legumes, grains, nuts and seeds which have mostly complex carbohydrates.

Fiber Can Make a Difference

Fiber, known as roughage, is an undigestible type of complex carbohydrate which has no nutritional value but helps to keep the intestinal tract in good working condition. Fiber is very helpful in lowering high cholesterol.

There are two forms of fiber. To get the benefits of both, you need to include both in your diet. Eating a variety of fiber-containing foods daily will help you get the amount of fiber you need. Although you require 20 to 30 grams of fiber daily, most Americans eat only approximately 10 grams daily.

Two forms of fiber:

1. Soluble--dissolves in water
2. Insoluble--does not dissolve in water

Soluble fiber

Soluble fiber dissolves in the fluids in the intestines but is not absorbed by the body. Pectin, certain gums and psyllium are soluble fibers. One of the gums is beta-glucan, which is present in oat products and beans and appears to be very beneficial in controlling cholesterol levels.

Approximately 10 to 25 grams of soluble fiber should be eaten daily. The highest concentration is found in:

- Rice bran
- Oat bran
- Rolled oats
- Barley
- Legumes (dried beans and peas, lentils)

- Fruits such as apples, applesauce, apricots, boysenberries, figs, pears, dried prunes
- Vegetables such as beets, broccoli, brussels sprouts, cabbage, carrots, corn, eggplant, lima beans, peas, potatoes with skin, zucchini

Soluble fiber makes a difference and helps:

- In lowering total cholesterol by lowering the "bad" LDL cholesterol
- Slow the absorption of glucose
- Control appetite by creating feeling of fullness

That soluble fiber aids in lowering cholesterol was first reported by Dr. James W. Anderson in 1977 at the University of Kentucky. He found that when a large amount of oat bran was eaten, the liver produced more bile acids, helping to remove cholesterol from the body through elimination. The liver also produced less cholesterol.

Rice bran is richer in soluble fiber than oat bran; two tablespoons of rice bran have as much soluble fiber as one-half cup of oat bran. Adding two tablespoons of rice bran or one-half cup of oat bran to your diet daily will help in lowering your cholesterol. Rice bran can be sprinkled right from the package on top of cereals, yogurt or fruit.

Dried beans and peas are another excellent source of soluble fiber which are able to be used in a wide variety of dishes.

You can increase your soluble fiber intake by eating:

- More vegetables and fruits high in soluble fiber
- Homemade bean and lentil dishes
- Oat bran and rice bran added to other foods
- Oatmeal and oat bran cereal
- Homemade oat and/or oat bran muffins

SOLUBLE FIBER[1] CONTENTS OF VARIOUS FOODS

Food Item 3½ oz. (100 Grams)	Soluble Fiber Grams	Food Item 3½ oz. (100 Grams)	Soluble Fiber Grams
Cereals		**Vegetables** continued	
All-Bran	0.0	Corn	1.1
Bran Buds	0.9	Cucumbers	0.9
Cornflakes	3.4	Eggplant	0.9
Cracked wheat	0.4	Green peppers	0.0
Farina	0.1	Kale, cooked	0.8
Grape-Nuts	0.2	Lettuce	0.6
Grits	3.3	Mushrooms	0.9
Oat bran	9.2	Onions, raw	1.0
Rolled oats	3.0	Onions, cooked	0.8
Rice bran	7.0	Parsnips	0.5
Shredded wheat	0.4	Peas, cooked	2.4
Wheat flakes	0.4	Potatoes, sweet; cooked	2.2
		Potatoes, white; cooked	2.0
Flours & Breads		Radishes	0.5
Rye flour, light	0.3	Rice, brown; cooked	0.0
Rye flour, dark	0.4	Rice, white; cooked	0.0
White flour	0.1	Spaghetti	0.1
Whole wheat flour	0.3	Spinach	1.4
Graham crackers, plain	0.3	Squash, summer; raw	1.4
Rye crackers	0.3	Squash, summer; cooked	1.0
Saltine crackes	0.1	Squash, white; cooked	0.3
Corn muffin	0.9	Tomatoes, raw	0.4
Oat bran muffin	3.0	Tomatoes, cooked	0.3
Whole wheat muffin	0.1	Turnips	1.0
Corn bread	1.1	Zucchini	1.4
French bread	0.1		
Rye bread	0.3	**Fruits**	
White bread	0.1	Apple	2.0
Whole wheat bread	0.3	Applesauce	0.8
		Apple juice	0.1
Vegetables		Apricots	1.0
Asparagus, raw	0.5	Apricots, canned	0.8
Asparagus, cooked	0.4	Banana	0.9
Barley, dry	0.4	Blackberries	0.9
Beans, green; cooked	0.8	Cherries	0.4
Beans, kidney; cooked	0.5	Cranberry juice	0.0
Beans, lima	0.4	Grapes	0.2
Beans, pinto	1.0	Grape juice	0.0
Bean sprouts, mung	0.6	Grapefruit	0.9
Beans, white; cooked	0.5	Lemon juice	0.0
Beet, cooked	0.9	Muskmelon	0.3
Broccoli	2.1	Orange	0.6
Brussels sprouts, cooked	0.9	Orange juice	0.3
Cabbage, raw	1.7	Peach	0.7
Cabbage, cooked	1.4	Peaches, canned	1.6
Carrots, raw	2.5	Pear	0.6
Carrots, cooked	1.4	Pears, canned	0.3
Cauliflower, raw	0.5	Pineapple	0.3
Cauliflower, cooked	0.3	Plum	1.0
Celery, raw	0.8	Strawberries	0.8
Celery, cooked	0.6	Tangerine	1.6

[1] Meat, milk and milk products contain no soluble fiber.

Insoluble fiber

Insoluble fiber does not dissolve in water and is not absorbed from the digestive tract. It is the fiber that gives plants their stability and structure.

Insoluble fiber is found in:

- Whole grains
- Wheat and corn bran
- Legumes
- Nuts
- Most fruits
- Most vegetables
- Seeds

Insoluble fiber makes a very big difference by:

- Speeding up the time it takes for food to move through the digestive tract, it is the ultimate in natural laxatives.
- Controlling the appetite by creating a feeling of fullness.
- Preventing diseases of digestive system such as diverticulosis, constipation and hemorrhoids and possibly colon cancer.

Additional aspects to consider

When beginning to add fiber to your diet, do it gradually if your digestive system is not accustomed to it because you may have increased flatulence (gas). Some people may experience cramping or mild diarrhea. These problems will lessen and disappear as your digestive system adjusts to the increased fiber. Constipation should be a problem of the past; your regularity will be improved and bowel movements will be large and soft and possibly more frequent. It is important that you drink six to eight 8 oz. glasses of water daily. Your ultimate goal could be to begin your day with a bowl of high fiber, low sugar cereal or homemade high fiber, low sugar muffins and end it with a delicious dried bean dish or lentil soup.

It is important for you to increase the amount of complex carbohydrates you eat so that you will get the fiber you need. The carbohydrates will also make up for the calories you will be losing as a result of eating less saturated fat. If you do not make up the lost calories, you may lose valuable nutrients, energy, and weight.

Foods you should eat more of to increase the complex carbohydrates in your diet:

- Dried beans and peas, lentils
- Whole grain products
- Vegetables, raw and cooked without cream sauces or gravies
- Fruits and unsweetened juices, consume more fresh whole fruit than juices

While adding more complex carbohydrates to your diet, be watchful that you do not consume more calories than your body requires to meet your needs. An excessive intake of calories, especially from heavily sugary and starchy foods tends to elevate your triglycerides. Alcoholic beverages are very high in calories and are poor bargains for calories since they have no food value. A word to the wise is, a careful selection of foods, with moderation, and no alcohol of any kind.

Remember: Complex carbohydrate foods, if eaten plain, are low in saturated fat and have no cholesterol. Many have soluble fiber. Sounds like a ticket to the world of ideal foods!

The following carbohydrate foods should be avoided because they are high in calories and/or saturated fat:

- Bakery products (cookies, croissants, sweet rolls, biscuits, muffins, cornbread)
- Granola cereals--usually high in fats
- Pastries

- Potato chips, or any chips made with fat
- Fried foods
- Refined sugars

4. Consider use of plant stanols/sterols found in such products as benacol and take control

Benacol and Take Control are vegetable oil spreads that can be used in place of butter or margarine. They are low in fat and the stanols and sterols in them are helpful in lowering LDL cholesterol. Because of the stanols and sterols these spreads could be considered as medication. Only two or three tablespoonsful are suggested to be used daily.

Benacol and Take Control cannot be used for cooking but can be used in any other way that butter or margarine would be used.

Calories from carbohydrates, proteins, and fats eaten in excess of immediate energy needs are converted to triglycerides. High levels of triglycerides are related to the development of atherosclerosis.

Summary and very brief review of food changes

This very brief review is the most pertinent information you need to remember and use concerning the foods to eat when controlling your cholesterol levels.

- Eat less total fat, especially saturated fat, found mostly in meats, dairy products, solid shortenings, and bakery goods
- When cooking and baking:

    Do not use saturated fats--solid shortenings, lard, butter, etc.

    Decrease polyunsaturated fats--most vegetable oils

    Increase monounsaturated fats--canola and olive oils

- Eat less quantities of foods containing cholesterol, found only in animal products

- Eat more complex carbohydrates, especially soluble fiber foods--oat bran, oatmeal, rice bran, vegetables, whole grains, legumes and fruits

B. Increase Physical Activity

This is the second of the three Therapeutic Lifestyle Changes that should be applied for improving your cholesterol levels. The first was the TLC diet, remember? Both changes are equal in their importance, one without the other is like putting on only one shoe. Authorities on cholesterol management have well established that doing both is very important for reaching that balance you should be striving for in improving your cholesterol levels.

Physical inactivity is a major underlying risk factor for CHD. It increases the lipid(fat) and nonlipid risk factors of the metabolic syndrome (see chapter two). It may also increase risk by impairing cardiovascular fitness and heart blood flow.

Rather than being physically inactive, become physically active for at least 30 minutes daily and reduce the risk of developing or dying from CHD or stroke.

Benefits of physical activity

Various studies have demonstrated that moderate regular physical activity can:

- Increase the good HDLs--age has no effect on the benefit but if you smoke, you may not receive the benefit
- Decrease triglycerides
- Lower LDLs
- Lower VLDLs
- Lower blood pressure
- Reduce insulin resistance
- Reduce stress, anxiety and depression
- Help weight control
- Improve cardiovascular function

One of the most interesting aspects of vigorous physical activity seldom gets any notice except by the body itself. As a result of exercising regularly, a network of small blood vessels (collateral circulation) in the heart muscle is increased and the coronary arteries open more. This allows more blood to reach the heart cells, delivering a greater supply of oxygen and nutrients. Another benefit is, if one of the coronary arteries is obstructed, the collateral circulation will still deliver blood to the area that is obstructed and less heart muscle damage will occur.

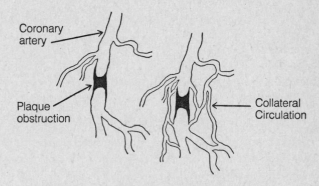

Increase of collateral circulation in coronary artery resulting from vigorous activity

Make physical activity a regular part of your daily routine

Choose activities that you enjoy and can and will do regularly. Some of you will prefer activities that fit into your daily routine, such as:

- walking with spouse, friends, children, pets, etc.
- using stairs instead of elevator or escalator
- housework
- gardening - digging, pulling weeds, etc.

- yardwork - use push mower, rake leaves
- playing with children
- taking extra trips up and down stairs
- parking at far end of parking lot rather than near the store entrance
- get off bus a few stops early and walk the remaining distance
- dancing

Others will prefer more vigorous activities including:

- brisk walking
- hiking
- jogging
- swimming
- canoeing
- bicycling - outdoor and stationary
- roller skating
- jumping rope
- tennis
- golf - pull cart or carry clubs
- dynamic dancing
- cross-country skiing

The above activities will increase your heart beat and produce beneficial changes in your respiratory and circulatory systems. Physical activity is most effective for the cardiovascular system if done in a rhythmic, repetitive manner. While doing your activity, you should be able to talk, if you cannot then you are working too hard and need to slow down or do something different.

Check That Pulse

In order for your physical activity to be considered vigorous, your pulse rate should increase to a certain point. See the chart below Pulse rates at rest vary among individuals due to personal traits and physical activities. It is not uncommon among athletes to have an at rest pulse rate as low as 40 beats a minute. These athletes would not need or be able to raise their rate to those in the chart below. To be prudent, check with your doctor to find out what your pulse rate should increase to when doing vigorous activities.

PULSE RATE DURING EXERCISE

AGE	PULSE RATE
20	120-150 beats per minute
25	117-146 beats per minute
30	114-142 beats per minute
35	111-138 beats per minute
40	108-135 beats per minute
45	105-131 beats per minute
50	102-127 beats per minute
55	99-123 beats per minute
60	96-120 beats per minute
65	93-116 beats per minute
70	90-113 beats per minute

Source: U.S. Department of Health and Human Services

To take your pulse, place your index and middle fingers of one hand on the artery in your wrist at the base of your thumb on the other hand. Count the beats for 15 seconds and multiply times 4 to get your pulse rate (heart beat) per minute.

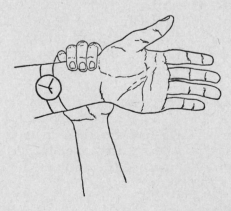

Talk To Your Doctor

Many adults will not need to see their doctors before becoming more physically active. But, if you are planning vigorous activities and have one or more of the following conditions, then check with your doctor before beginning:

- Health condition such as:
  coronary heart disease
  high blood pressure
  diabetes
  osteoporosis
  obesity
- High risk for coronary heart disease
- Over age 40 for men
- Over age 50 for women

Reviewing your various activity options with your doctor can help you select an activity well suited to your age and physical condition. If you plan to do vigorous activity, you may need a stress test before you can determine the activity best suited for you. Your activity should challenge your circulatory system at an intensity that's appropriate for you.

If you are recovering from a heart attack or heart surgery, your doctor may suggest you begin your physical activity program in a cardiac rehabilitation center. During your activity either at the center or at home, if you experience discomfort in your chest, neck, arms or surrounding area; feel faint or light-headed; or become extremely out of breath, stop the activity at once and contact your physician as soon as possible. Don't wait until severe pain occurs before seeing your doctor.

Special Things To Remember

No matter what type or degree of activity you choose, the important idea is to do at least moderately physical activity everyday for a minimum of 30 minutes. If you can't find time to do 30 minutes or more at one time, then divide the time into 2 or 3 segments.

After you decide your physical activity, it is important to:

- Know your limits, begin slowly and gradually increase the intensity and duration over the weeks.
- Always ease into (warm up) and out of (cool down) your exercise. Do five minutes of flexing and slowly running in place at the beginning and five minutes of walking and stretching at the end of your exercise.
- Dress appropriately and wear the proper footwear.
- Exercise only on a flexible surface, never on concrete, etc.
- Do not exercise for at least one hour after a meal.

When making the transition from inactivity to vigorous activity, warming up with flexing exercises is important for reducing the strain on muscles, joints and ligaments. The warm up allows for gradual circulatory adjustment and increases in muscle temperature, reducing the chances of orthopedic injury and heightening muscle efficiency and oxygen exchange between blood and tissues.

It is equally important to make a gradual transition from vigorous activity to non-activity. The cool down prevents a rapid fall in blood pressure which might cause fainting, irregular heart rhythms, or more serious complications. Blood vessels dilate in exercising muscles. If exercise is ended abruptly, especially if you stand motionless after exercise, there may be a fall in your blood pressure, pooling of blood in the veins and a decreased return of blood to the heart and brain. If you cool down by walking and stretching, your circulatory system has a chance to adjust to your new level of activity and keep your blood moving to all parts of your body.

So the next time you see someone going through all those contortions before or after exercising, you now know it's not "show biz," it's simply someone knowing and doing the correct thing.

Do not take a shower, steam bath or sauna immediately after exercising because the heat from them can put too much of a burden on your circulatory system. You must wait until your internal heat, which was increased by exercise, can be lessened and your circulation restored to normal.

Be sure the physical activity is one that you will enjoy and can be done easily and year round in the area where you live. If these factors are met, you will be much more likely to be physically active frequently.

Attention!!!
Your children over 2 years of age should be tested if either of the biological parents has or ever had a high cholesterol (above 240).

C. Weight Management

This is the third of the three Therapeutic Lifestyle Changes (TLC). The first was the TLC diet and the second was increase physical activity. Weight management is as important as the TLC diet and physical activity. All three work together to create an effect which magically helps to bring your cholesterol numbers to where they should be. So rub Aladdin's lamp and let the magic begin.

Overweight and obesity are recognized as major underlying risk factors for CHD because individuals with these conditions frequently have:

- High levels of "bad" LDL cholesterol
- High levels of triglycerides
- Low levels of the "good" HDL cholesterol
- High blood pressure
- High fasting blood glucose

The potential benefits of weight reduction are:

- Lower LDL cholesterol level
- Lower triglycerides level

- Higher HDL cholesterol level
- Lower blood pressure
- Lower fasting blood glucose

Weight management includes the reduction of excess weight and maintenance of this lower body weight. There are two ways besides actual weight to relate to excess body weight, these are:

1. Body mass index (BMI)
2. Waist circumference

1. Body mass index (BMI)

The BMI is a measure of your weight relative to your height. This is a good indicator of your risk for a variety of diseases since it gives an accurate estimate of your total body fat. The BMI gives you a more precise evaluation of body fat than weight alone. You can determine your BMI by a couple of simple calculations.

Use for pounds and inches measurements:

BMI = weight (pounds) x 703 divided by height in inches squared ($inches^2$)

Example: Person is 5 feet 5 inches tall and weighs 180 lbs.

1. Multiply weight in pounds by 703.......180 x 703 = 126,540

2. Divide the answer in step 1 by height in inches squared (65 x 65 = 4225)..................................126,540 ÷ 4225 = 29.9

Use for metric system

BMI = weight (kg) divided by height squared (m^2)

Meaning of BMI Number

Underweight	less than 18.5
Normal	18.5 - 24.9
Overweight	25 - 29.9
Obesity	30 and above

2. Waist circumference

Waist circumference is a way to evaluate abdominal fat before and during weight loss. Abdominal fat is associated with a greater health risk, especially for CHD and diabetes, than peripheral fat such as in the buttocks-thigh area. Determine your waist circumference by placing a measuring tape snugly around your waist.

Waist measurement should be:

female - less than 35 inches (less than 88 cm)
male - less than 40 inches (less than 102 cm)

If you are overweight (BMI 25 to 29.9), but you do not have a high waist measurement, and have less than 2 risk factors, it's important that you not gain additional weight.

If you are overweight (BMI 25 to 29.9) and have 2 or more risk factors, or if you are obese (BMI 30 or more), it is very important that you lose weight.

Risk factors:

- high blood pressure (hypertension)
- high LDL-cholesterol ("bad" cholesterol)
- low HDL-cholesterol ("good" cholesterol)
- high triglycerides
- high blood glucose (sugar)
- family history of premature heart disease
- physical inactivity
- cigarette smoking

If you need to lose weight, there are no quick fixes. There are three things you will need to address:

1. Eat less calories daily
2. Do moderate to intense physical activity everyday
3. Modify your behavior

The initial goal of weight loss should be to reduce body weight by about 10 percent from your present weight. With success, and if warranted, further weight loss can be attempted. Weight loss should be about 1 to 2 pounds per week for a period of 6 months which makes it easier to keep off.

1. Eat less calories daily

To achieve or maintain a recommended weight, your daily caloric intake must not exceed the number of calories your body burns daily. Therefore if you eat fewer calories and increase your physical activity on a regular basis, you should reduce your weight. It is suggested not to decrease your daily calorie intake below what is recommended for your desired weight, for your age and height, see chart below. It is best to work with your doctor when losing weight; he/she may advise you to speak with a dietician or nutritionist as well.

Calories say, "Not all foods are equal"

Plan well-balanced meals and snacks around familiar foods. Avoid or limit highly starchy foods (pasta, rice, corn, potatoes, etc) and sugary foods. Substitute complex carbohydrates (whole grains, vegetables, fruits) for high-fat and high calorie foods. Remember, fat has nine calories per gram weight whereas carbohydrate and protein have only four calories per gram weight. What better case could you have for showing, "Not all foods are equal."

RECOMMENDED DAILY CALORIE ALLOWANCE

	Age	Wt.	Ht.	Calories
Males	19-22	147 lb.	69	3000
	23-50	154	69	2700
	51+	154	69	2400
Females	19-22	128 lb.	65	2100
	23-50	128	65	2000
	51+	128	65	1800

Source: Food and Nutrition Board, National Academy of Science/National Research Council

Ways to reduce the amount of calories eaten

Reducing the amount of fat you eat is a practical way to reduce calories. But reducing fat intake alone without reducing calories is not sufficient for weight loss. However, reducing fat, along with reducing carbohydrates can help reduce calories. You need to remember that it is not only what you eat but also how much you eat that's important. Be familiar with serving sizes for various foods, such as:

- 1 serving of fruit = whole medium apple, banana, or orange; $1/2$ grapefruit; a wedge of melon; $3/4$ cup fruit juice; $1/2$ cup berries; $1/2$ cup chopped fresh, cooked or canned fruit; $1/4$ cup dried fruit.

- 1 serving of vegetables = $1/2$ cup cooked or chopped raw vegetables; 1 cup leafy raw vegetables, such as lettuce or spinach; $1/2$ cup cooked beans or other legumes; $3/4$ cup vegetable juice.

- 1 serving of meat = 2 to 3 oz. of cooked lean meat, poultry without skin or fish.

- 1 serving of milk, yogurt, cheese = 1 cup milk, 8 oz. yogurt, 1 oz. hard cheese, $1/2$ cup cottage cheese.

- 1 serving of cooked rice, potato and cereal = $1/2$ cup.

- 1 serving of bread = 1 slice, $1/2$ hamburger roll or English muffin, 1 small roll, biscuit or muffin.

Look for size of serving on packaged foods - frozen and canned fruits, vegetables and soups.

Since you usually aren't going to be measuring everything you eat, there are a couple of things you can do to get an eyeball measurement.

1. For later mental reference, you can actually measure some foods to see what 2 to 3 oz. of cooked meat and $1/2$, $3/4$ and 1 cup measure of various foods look like.

2. Use your hand to approximate serving size.

- Palm of your hand or a deck of cards is approximately the size of 3 oz. of meat, fish or poultry.
- Cupped hand can hold approximately 2 oz. of nuts.
- Fist is about a cup, so $1/2$ of fist is serving for mashed potatoes, cooked rice, pasta and cereal.
- Thumb from tip to second joint is about an ounce of cheese.
- Tip of thumb is about a teaspoon (3 tips = tablespoon), good for measuring jelly, peanut butter, soft vegetable oil spreads.

Some other tips:

- Use smaller plate from which to eat - moderate servings won't appear small.

- Only eat when sitting at a table - this helps avoid "tasting" while preparing foods.

- Eat slowly - it takes about 20 minutes after you begin eating for the feeling of fullness or satisfaction to occur. Eating slowly will help you feel full before you have overeaten.

- Drink a glass of water before eating - it helps you reach the full (satisfied) feeling.

- Beginning a meal with broth-based soup can help you feel fuller.

- Avoid watching TV or reading while eating.

- Eat raw vegetables and fruit for snacks - have them prepared ahead of time so you can just reach in the refrigerator for them.

- Only buy what you should be eating, not extra to have on hand just in case of company.

- Use low fat versions of high fat foods.

2. Do moderate to intense physical activity daily

A key concept to remember and use is; 3500 calories equals 1 lb of weight gain or loss. Consider depleting 3500 calories a week by a combination of eating fewer calories and burning up calories through physical activity. A practical approach is to target 500 calories daily (500 cal. x 7 days = 3500 cal.) by eating less and being more physically active. This could lead to a one pound loss per week.

A slow method of losing weight is the healthiest approach and has the longest lasting benefit. Weight should be reduced over a long, not short, period of time.

ESTIMATED CALORIES BURNED BY AVERAGE 150 LB. PERSON EXERCISING 1 HOUR	
Activity	Calories burned
Bicycling	240-420
Cross-country skiing	600
Dancing	240-420
Housework	100
Jogging, 5 1/2 mph	660
Jogging, 7 mph	920
Jumping rope	750
Rowing	250-420
Running in place	650
Swimming, 25 yds/min	275
Swimming, 50 yds/min	500
Tennis, singles	420
Walking, 2 mph	240
Walking, 3 mph	320

Examples of moderate amounts* of physical activity ranging from less vigorous/more time to more vigorous/less time.

Common Chores	Sporting Activities
Washing and waxing a car for 45-60 minutes	Playing volleyball for 45 - 60 minutes
Washing windows or floors for 45-60 minutes	Playing touch football for 45 minutes
Gardening for 30-45 minutes	Walking 1 3/4 miles in 35 minute (20 min/mile)
Wheeling self in wheel-chair 30-40 minutes	Basketball (shooting baskets) 30 minutes
Pushing a stroller 1 1/2 miles in 30 minutes	Bicycling 5 miles in 30 minutes
Raking leaves for 30 minutes	Dancing fast (social) for 30 minutes
Walking 2 miles in 30 minutes (15 min/mile)	Water aerobics for 30 minutes
Shoveling snow for 15 minutes	Swimming Laps for 20 minutes
Stairwalking for 15 minutes.	Play basketball for 15-20 mins. Jumping rope for 15 minutes Running 1 1/2 miles in 15 min. (10 min/mile)

Source: NHLBI Obesity Education Initiative

* A moderate amount of physical activity is roughly equivalent to physical activity that uses approximately 150 calories of energy per day, or 1,000 calories per week.

By following the food and exercise suggestions in this chapter, you should be able to achieve your desirable weight, see following charts.

DESIRABLE WEIGHT FOR HEIGHT CHART

Men age 25 and over*

height (1" heels)	small frame	medium frame	large frame
5' 2"	112-120	118-129	126-141
4 3	115-123	121-133	129-144
5 4	118-126	124-136	132-148
5 5	121-129	127-139	135-152
5 6	124-133	130-143	138-156
5 7	128-137	134-147	142-161
5 8	132-141	138-152	147-166
5 9	136-145	142-156	151-170
5 10	140-150	146-160	155-174
5 11	144-154	150-165	159-179
6 0	148-158	154-170	164-184
6 1	152-162	158-175	168-189
6 2	156-167	162-180	173-194
6 3	160-171	167-185	178-199
6 4	164-175	172-190	182-204

DESIRABLE WEIGHT FOR HEIGHT CHART

Women age 25 and over*

height (2" heels)	small frame	medium frame	large frame
4' 10"	92-98	96-107	104-119
4 11	94-101	98-110	106-122
5 0	96-104	101-113	109-125
5 1	99-107	104-116	112-128
5 2	102-110	107-119	115-131
5 3	105-113	110-122	118-134
5 4	108-116	113-126	121-138
5 5	111-119	116-130	125-142
5 6	114-123	120-135	129-146
5 7	118-127	124-139	133-150
5 8	122-131	128-143	137-154
5 9	126-135	132-147	141-158
5 10	130-140	136-151	145-163
5 11	134-144	140-155	149-168
6 0	138-148	144-159	153-173

* Weight in pounds according to frame (in indoor clothing). For nude weight, deduct 5 to 7 lb. Information prepared by Metropolitan Life Insurance Company.

3. Modify your behavior

Sometimes problems and situations can be resolved simply by changing how you are processing the information. If you change how you think about an issue, you can alter how you react to the situation and solve the problem.

Rather than focus on weight loss, focus on dietary and physical activity changes which will be much more productive.

Setting goals is a good idea as long as the goals are:

- specific
- realistic
- flexible

For example:
Be more "physically active" is a good goal but it is not specific enough.

"Walk 4 miles every day" is specific and measurable, but probably not realistic if you are just beginning.

"Walk 30 minutes every day" is more realistic, but what happens if you're not able to walk on a couple of days due to unforeseen conditions?

"Walk 30 minutes, 5 days a week" is specific, realistic and flexible.

Set some short term goals that get you closer and closer by small steps to the ultimate goal such as eating less fat. Reduce your intake of fat from 40% to 35% and finally to 30% of your total daily calories. This is based on the idea that nothings succeeds like success.

When you reach goals, reward yourself, but not with food. An effective reward is something that is desirable, timely and dependent upon meeting your goal. A reward might be something material or an act of self-kindness.

Frequent small rewards are usually more effective than larger rewards that involve a long time period. For example, how about queen or king for the day at the local spa or an evening for yourself to just read or relax.

Observing and recording your weight regularly is key to keeping it off. Remember the four following concepts:

1. One day's food intake and physical activity won't necessarily affect your weight the next day. Your weight will change quite a bit over the course of a few days because of fluctuations in water and bodyfat.

2. Try to weigh yourself at a set time once or twice per week.

3. Whatever time you choose to weigh yourself, make certain it is always the same time, the same scale and be dressed in similar clothing.

4. May be helpful to create a graph of your weight as a visual aide of your progress rather than just listing numbers.

Learn what social or environmental signals encourage undesired eating and then alter or remove those entrapping signals. Some signals for overeating or eating undesirable foods may be:

• Watching TV or going to a movie

• Driving past donut shops and fast food stores

• Coffee breaktime at work-snacks at coffee pot

• Certain people

Come up with ways to:

• Separate the association of eating with certain signals.

- Avoid or eliminate the signal - don't drive by a donut or fast food store, ask someone to bring you coffee at breaktime.

- Change environment - meet friends in noneating places such as your home, concerts, parks, museums, etc.

To achieve or maintain a recommended weight be certain to:

- Have a sense of commitment - do what you need to do.
- Review your eating habits - keep a food journal.
- Compare how many calories you eat daily with the amount you should be eating daily.
- Eat only the number of calories needed for maintaining your desirable weight, not for losing weight.
- Have sufficient physical activity to burn up any excess calories and/or weight.

Helpful tips for reducing your weight:

- Eat three meals a day at regular times.
- Don't skip meals, it lowers your resistance to snacking between meals which may equal more calories in the end.
- Relax and sit at a table whenever you eat.
- Put food portion on your plate and don't have seconds.
- Concentrate on enjoying your food, don't watch TV or read while you eat.
- Have raw vegetables and fruits handy for quality snacks rather than high-calorie snacks and junk food.
- Avoid fast foods, usually high in fat; instead, eat from the salad bar.
- Go grocery shopping only after you have eaten, not when you are hungry.
- Avoid all alcohol--ounce for ounce, it has almost as many calories as fat. Use mineral water with a slice of lemon or lime.
- Walk rather than ride and use stairs rather than elevator or escalator when possible.

Remember, if you are having any difficulty with either maintaining or reducing your weight, you are probably taking in too many calories in relation to your physical activity. Once again you must realize that no plan works better than the way you have organized and managed it.

SUMMARY OF FOLLOWING THE THERAPEUTIC LIFESTYLE CHANGES	
Doing this	*Results in*
Eat more monounsaturated fats (canola and olive oils)	Lower LDL cholesterol level
Eat less saturated fat	Lower LDL cholesterol level
Eat less calories, reduce weight	Lower triglyceride level
Increase physical activity	Higher HDL cholesterol level

Additional Things That May Improve Your Cholesterol Numbers

In most cases, the three Therapeutic Lifestyle Changes are the only necessary changes needed to improve your cholesterol numbers. However, there are additional things you can do that may help your cholesterol reach more beneficial levels.

Stop smoking, stop drinking coffee and alcohol

In this day and age it seems absurd to have to say, "don't smoke and don't drink coffee or alcohol!" Although there are still some unanswered questions about coffee and alcohol, the show is closed when it comes to smoking. It is just a matter of time until the scientific world will bring down the curtain on coffee and alcohol as well. A health conscious person doesn't need to see act three and the curtain come down before stopping coffee and alcohol.

Studies have shown that:

- Smoking lowers your "good" HDLs and raises your "bad" LDLs.

- Coffee may raise your LDL cholesterol, triglycerides and lower your "good" HDLs.
- Alcohol in a small quantity may have some very limited benefit, but that benefit is far outweighed by all of the negative aspects of alcohol consumption. To increase your life's overall benefits, don't drink alcohol at all.

MEDICATIONS FOR CONTROLLING YOUR CHOLESTEROL

If medication is prescribed for you, you will also need to follow the TLC and control your other risk factors for CHD such as:

- smoking
- high blood pressure
- diabetes

Doing all of the above may decrease the amount of medication you require and/or help the medication work more effectively.

Medication for lowering LDL cholesterol will be considered when:

- CHD or heart disease risk equivalents are present.

- Short-term or long-term risk for CHD is high.

- After 3 months of lifestyle changes, LDL goal is not met

When your LDL goal is met, if your triglycerides are still high and/or your HDLs are low another type of medication may be given to you.

There are several types of medications used for improving your blood cholesterol:

1. Statins - lovastatin, pravastatin, simvastatin, atorvastatin, and cerivastatin. Statins lower LDL cholesterol more than

any other type of medication, help raise HDL cholesterol and lower triglycerides.

2. Bile acid sequestrants - cholestyramine, colestipol and coleseveam. Lower LDL cholesterol and raise HDL cholesterol a little.

3. Nicotinic acid(niacin) a B vitamin - Lowers LDL cholesterol and triglycerides and raises HDL cholesterol.

4. Fibric acids - gemfibrozil, fenofibrate, clofibrate. Used mostly to lower triglycerides and raise HDL cholesterol a small amount.

If placed on medication, be certain your doctor explains:

- Exactly how and when it is to be taken (before, with or after meals).
- All the side effects and what to do about them.
- With which medical conditions the medications should not be used.
- Its interactions with other medications, foods or alcohol.
- How long to take the medication.
- If periodic blood tests are necessary.
- If there will be any interference with regular activities, such as exercise or sexual.
- What to do if you forget a dose of medication.

In the event you are advised to use medication, you should:

1. Go to your local library and ask the reference librarian for the books titled:
   - AMA Drug Evaluation '
   - United States Pharmacopeia Drug Information For The Consumer

   These books list medications and give the manufactures' information including contraindication, side effects, etc. You may want to copy the pertinent details to review at your leisure.

2. Ask your pharmacist for the information sheet that comes with the medication.

3. Learn the names and doses of all your medications.

4. Do not suddenly stop taking you medication; this can be dangerous because some medication need to be tapered off gradually. Consult first with your doctor before making any changes in taking your medication.

It is your personal responsibility as a patient and a consumer to know as much as possible about the substances you are taking into your body. Your doctor is your helper in maintaining your wellness, but it is your responsibility to take the primary interest when he/she is trying to help you. Don't just throw yourself at your physician's feet and whine; take some initiative and responsibility. You must stay responsible for your own personal well being and not just rely on other people helping you.

If you have a medical condition such as diabetes, gout, liver disease, peptic ulcer, renal disease, etc., you must be certain your physician is aware of it before placing you on any cholesterol lowering medication. Some cholesterol lowering medications are not compatible with the above or other conditions.

CHOLESTEROL LOWERING PROGRESS CHART

Have Total Lipid
Profile Test
↓
Results:
Elevated LDL
↓
Your Physician sets
Your LDL goals
↓
Begin TLC in Chapter Four
↓
After 6 weeks have blood test for LDL level
↓
Has your LDL goal been met?
↓

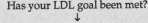

↓	↓
Yes	No
↓	↓
Continue what you have been doing	Eat less saturated fat and cholesterol
↓	Increase fiber intake
In 4 to 6 months check with your doctor for long term follow-up	Consider adding plant stanols/sterols
	Consider consulting nutritionist
	↓

After 6 weeks have blood test for LDL level
↓
Has your LDL goal been met
↓

↓	↓
Yes	No
↓	↓
Continue what you have been doing	Medication may be considered
↓	Intensify weight management and physical activity
In 4 to 6 months check with your doctor for long-term follow-up	Consider consulting nutritionist
	↓
	Check with doctor every 6 weeks until goal is met

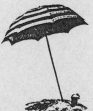

See you on the beach.
The umbrella is up;
you bring the chairs.

5

3 WEEK PLAN FOR CONTROLLING YOUR CHOLESTEROL

Three weeks is an ideal period of time in which to make the necessary transitions for improving your cholesterol levels and becoming accustomed to the food and physical activity adjustments. Some people, because of their lifestyles, personalities, etc. may take a little longer to make all the necessary transitions. So do not become discouraged; each positive effort has a benefit toward what you are trying to achieve.

The 3 Week Plan is a structured way to follow the food and physical activity information given in the previous chapter, How To Control Your Cholesterol, and is ideal for working with your doctor and dietician/nutritionist. The Plan does not list all of the foods to eat or to avoid but rather suggests foods high in soluble fiber and low in saturated fat which you should be using to replace foods high in saturated fats and cholesterol.

The quantity of food to eat is usually not given; you decide the quantity based on whether or not you need to reduce your weight. It is impossible to structure a plan that is suited to everyone's needs and tastes. Subsequently the 3 Week Plan is a foundation on which to build, according to your individual needs and tastes, using the information in the previous chapter. As always, the information should complement your doctor's recommendations.

THE GOAL OF THE 3 WEEK PLAN

The goal of the 3 Week Plan is to give you a structure for easing into your lifestyle changes.

During the three weeks you will:

Eat less:
- Saturated fat
- Total fat
- Cholesterol

Eat more:
- Complex carbohydrates--soluble fiber
- Monounsaturated fat

Do more:
- Physical activity

Attention!!!
Individuals who have CHD before the age of 55 may have children who have CHD risk factors that need attention.   See chapter, Cholesterol Concerns For Children and Adolescents.

THE METHOD OF THE 3 WEEK PLAN

When making dietary and physical activity changes, it is best to make the transitions slowly so that your body can adjust properly and the changes do not overwhelm you. Sample menus are included as examples of how you can make the food transition slowly. The sample menus are only examples, they are not chiseled in stone or bone. Physical activity is gradually increased by the week. Changes are made week by week.

Follow one week at a time.

1st Week--getting into position
2nd Week--moving along with additional modifications
3rd Week--locking in lifetime eating and activity habits

1st Week--Getting into Position

Modify shopping list:

2% milk rather than whole milk
Canola and/or olive oil rather than other vegetable oils
Oat bran cereal
Soft margarine, in place of butter, with no trans fatty acids and with acceptable vegetable oil listed first
Raisins
Canned or dried navy, kidney, pinto and garbanzo beans
Whole grain bread and crackers (Kavli, Ryvita, Finn Crisp, Rye Krisp or Wasa) if you eat bread and crackers
Natural peanut butter with no hydrogenated oil
Whole grain flour for baking if you bake
Nonstick cooking spray

Don't buy:

Commercially baked goods and crackers--high in fat and usually made with hydrogenated oils or palm or coconut oil
Ice cream
Prepared fried items such as chicken, fish, french fries etc.

Eat daily:

Oat bran cereal made with 1/3 cup oat bran
    or
1/2 cup cooked beans (navy, kidney or pinto)
    or
2 homemade oat bran muffins
1 serving fruit high in soluble fiber
8 eight ounce glasses of water

Do:

Use 2% milk
Use canola and/or olive oil in place of other vegetable oils
Use soft margarine rather than butter
Not eat fried foods
Decide what physical activity you plan to do and if necessary discuss with your doctor if it is appropriate for you
Begin increasing physical activity slowly

1st week sample menus - note: items with * are in cookbook section

Breakfast:
    orange juice
* oat bran cereal, made with 1/3 cup oat bran
    2% milk, 1/2 to 1 cup
    water, eight ounces

Snack: (optional)
    V-8 juice, 1/2 to 1 cup

Lunch:
    lean roast beef sandwich on whole grain bread
    tomato, lettuce & cucumber salad
    apple
    water, eight ounces

Snack: (optional)
    whole grain English muffin
    soft margarine, 2 tsp.

Dinner:
    chicken breast, baked
    corn
    cauliflower, sprinkled with grated parmesan cheese
    asparagus
    whole grain roll
    soft margarine, 1 tsp.
    fresh fruit cup
    water, eight ounces

Breakfast:
    1/2 grapefruit
    soft boiled egg
    whole grain toast, 1 to 2 slices
    soft margarine, 1 to 2 tsp.
    water, eight ounces

Snack: (optional)
    banana
    water, eight ounces

Lunch:
* oat bran muffins, 2
  soft margarine, 2 tsp.
  low fat cottage cheese, 1/2 cup
  crushed pineapple, 3 Tbs. mixed into cottage cheese
  carrot sticks
  water, eight ounces

Snack: (optional)
  1/4 cup raisins

Dinner:
  lean sirloin steak, 4 oz.
  baked potato with Butter Buds
  carrots with ginger
  green beans
  whole grain roll
  soft margarine, 1 tsp.
* angel food cake topped with fresh unsweetened fruit

Breakfast:
  grapefruit, 1/2
* french toast
  soft margarine, 2 tsp.
  fruit only preserves
  2% milk, 1 glass
  water, eight ounces

Snack: (optional)
  Rye Krisp crackers, 5
  2 tsp. natural peanut butter

Lunch:
  tomato juice, 1 glass
  tuna fish pita sandwich
  raw broccoli & cauliflower flowerets
  apple
  water, eight ounces

Snack: (optional)
   dried apricots, 4 or 5

Dinner:
* bean soup
   mixed vegetable salad
   whole grain bread
   margarine 2 tsp.
   tea, 1 cup
    water, eight ounces

2nd Week--Moving Along With Additional Modifications

Modify shopping list:
   Continue with 1st Week items
   1% milk rather than 2% milk
   Lean cuts of red meat--not prime or choice cuts
   Very lean ground beef
   Poultry
   Lentils
   Low fat cheeses and yogurt if you eat cheese and yogurt
   Lots of fruits and vegetables high in soluble fiber such as:
      prunes, apples, dried apricots, pears, figs, dates, citrus,
      broccoli, brussel sprouts, carrots, corn, lima beans
   Preserves with no added sugar
   Unsweetened applesauce

Don't buy:
   Continue with recommendations for 1st week
   Lunch meats
   Frozen vegetables with sauces or butter
   Whole milk products

Eat daily:
   Drink 8, eight ounce glasses of water
   2 servings of fruit high in soluble fiber
   2 servings of any of the following:
      Oat bran cereal, 1 cup cooked beans (chili, baked beans,
      bean soup), 1 home made oat bran muffins
   At least 1 serving of vegetable high in soluble fiber

Do:
  Continue with recommendations of 1st week
  Trim all visible fat from meat before and after cooking
  Remove skin from poultry before cooking
  Use 2 egg whites in place of each whole egg called for in
    recipes
  Use unsweetened applesauce in place of some of the oil in
    recipes for baked items, ie. 1/2 oil and 1/2 applesauce
  Use canola oil in place of solid shortening (butter, crisco, etc.)
    in recipes for baked items
  Use 1 % milk rather than 2% milk
  Eat only low fat dairy products--cheese, yogurt
  Use evaporated skim milk in place of cream or half & half
  Physical activity 5 days for 20 to 30 minutes

2nd week sample menus - note: items with * are in cookbook
section

Breakfast:
  stewed prunes
* oat pancakes
  margarine, 2 tsp.
  unsweetened applesauce or jam
  1% milk, 1/2 to 1 cup
   water, eight ounces

Snack: (optional)
  Kavali cracker with 2 tsp. peanut butter (natural, no hydrogenated oil)

Lunch:
  ham (3 1/2 oz) sandwich on whole grain bread
    with lettuce and tomato
  tart apple
  tea
   water, eight ounces

Snack: (optional)
* oat bran muffin with applesauce

Dinner:
* oven fried chicken teriyaki, skin removed
  corn
  spinach
  boiled potatoes with parsley
  margarine, 1 tsp.
  fresh strawberries
    water, eight ounces

Breakfast:
  orange cut in eighths
  * oat bran muffins, 2
  margarine, 2 tsp.
  1% milk, 1 glass
    water, eight ounces

Snack: (optional)
  peach

Lunch:
* lentil soup
  vegetable salad
  whole grain toast
  margarine, 2 tsp.
    water, eight ounces

Snack: (optional)
* soft strawberry ice cream

Dinner:
* turkey stroganoff
  noodles
  green beans
  carrots
  seedless grapes
    water, eight ounces

Breakfast:
  1/4 cantaloupe
* oat bran cereal
  1% milk, 1/2 to 1 cup
    water, eight ounces

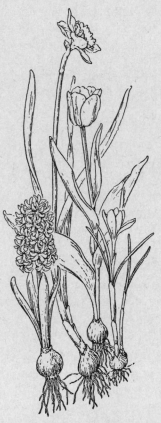

Snack: (optional)
lowfat plain yogurt with fresh fruit added (strawberries, banana, peach)

Lunch:
* turkey chili
salad
whole grain bread
margarine, 2 tsp.
* orange pineapple gelatin
water, eight ounces

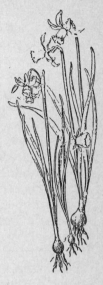

Snack:
Rye-Krisp cracker and low fat cheese

Dinner:
spaghetti with lean ground beef meat sauce
grated parmesan cheese, 3 Tbs.
* vegetable salad
whole grain French bread
baked apple
water, eight ounces

3rd Week--Locking in Lifetime Eating and Physical Activity Habits

Modify shopping list:
Continue with 1st and 2nd week items
Nonfat or skim milk rather than 1% milk
Tofu--soybean product
Fish and/or seafood
Light Salad Dressings and/or mayonnaise
Nonstick cooking spray
Ground turkey and/or chicken breast
Turkey or chicken breast cutlets
Barley
Rice bran
Cornmeal

Don't buy:
Continue with recommendations for 1st and 2nd weeks
Prepared soups--usually high in fat and salt

Eat daily:
Drink 8 eight ounce glasses of water
3 servings of fruit high in soluble fiber
At least 2 servings of vegetables high in soluble fiber
1 serving of oat bran cereal or cooked beans or lentils or home made bran muffins

Do:
Continue with recommendations for 1st & 2nd weeks
Eat fish or seafood
Eat ground turkey or chicken breasts rather than ground beef
Eat 2 meatless meals a week
Use light mayonnaise and/or mustard on sandwiches rather than butter or margarine
Use light dressings on salads
Use only sugarless jam or jelly rather than margarine on breads and muffins
Eat whole grain bread, muffins and crackers rather than regular bread, muffins and crackers
Lessen the amount of sugar in your recipes; can usually be decreased by at least one half gradually. Increase the flavor extract (vanilla, lemon, etc) and spices (cinnamon, nutmeg, ginger, etc).
Physical activity 6 - 7 days for at least 30 to 40 minutes

3rd week sample menus - note: items with * are in cookbook section

Breakfast:
*banana breakfast drink, made with skim milk
corn muffin, 2
unsweetened jelly or applesauce
water, eight ounces

Snack: (optional)
dried apricots

Lunch:
* lentil soup
  salad
  whole grain bread or toast with unsweetened jam
  low fat frozen yogurt
  water, eight ounces

Snack: (optional)
  raw vegetables
  toasted plain corn tortilla

Dinner:
  shrimp Creole
  brown rice
  cheesy zucchini
  spinach salad
  seasonal fruit cup
   water, eight ounces

Breakfast:
  fresh pineapple
* oat pancakes
  unsweetened applesauce
  skim milk, 1 glass
   water, eight ounces

Snack: (optional)
  apple

Lunch:
  lowfat cottage cheese with fresh fruit
  whole grain muffin, 2
  celery & carrot sticks
  tea
   water, eight ounces

Snack: (optional)
  air-popped popcorn

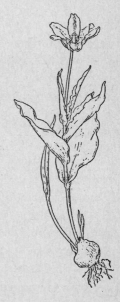

Dinner:
  broiled salmon
  rice
  margarine, 2 tsp.
  snow peas, steamed
  beets
  Sorbet
  water, eight ounces

Breakfast:
  orange cut in eighths
  oatmeal with 2 Tbs. raisins
  skim milk,　1/2 to 1 cup
   water, eight ounces

Snack: (optional)
  lowfat plain yogurt with applesauce and cinnamon added

Lunch:
* minestrone soup
* oat bran muffins
  unsweetened applesauce
  tea
  water, eight ounces

Snack: (optional)
  pear

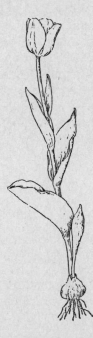

Dinner:
  ground turkey breast meatloaf
  baked potato
  brussel sprouts
  lima beans
  Angle food cake
  water, eight ounces

LIFETIME LIFESTYLE

For the rest of your life follow the 3rd week of the Plan with the following modifications.

Eat:
Fish 2 to 3 times a week
A meatless meal (tofu, beans, lentils, etc.) at least 2 to 3 times a week
Poultry 3 to 4 times a week
Very lean red meat no more than 2 or 3 times a week
Foods high in soluble fiber daily - fruits, vegetables, beans, legumes and whole grains

Snacks:
Air-popped popcorn
Whole grain crackers (Kavli, Ryvita, Finn Crisp, Rye Crisp or Wasa)
Fresh or dried fruit
Raw vegetables
*Soft strawberry ice cream
Home made oat bran muffin
Celery, apple or cracker with natural peanut butter - no hydrogenated oil
Low fat cheese
Low fat yogurt with fresh fruit
Vegetable juice

Do:
Physical activity for at least 30 to 45 minutes 5 - 7 days per week

DAILY FOOD REVIEW AND ACCOUNTING

Some individuals involved in the game plan of controlling their cholesterol find it useful to do a daily food intake review and accounting chart. If you are one of these individuals, we have supplied a blank chart (chart #3) at the end of this chapter which can be copied and used to list the foods you eat daily. You can then do an accounting of the total calories, fat, and cholesterol you have eaten for the day to see if you are within the recommended limits.

Also supplied, are a model chart for a "present" or "before" eating style and a model chart showing a "cholesterol lowering" or "after" eating style. If you compare the totals of these two charts, you will easily notice the differences in the fat, cholesterol, soluble fiber and calorie intake. Be sure to also note that in the cholesterol lowering chart, the foods are not dull or small in quantity.

You may want to complete a chart for the way you are presently eating and another for after you begin the cholesterol lowering Plan. After completing your charts, compare your total intake in the various columns with the recommendations given in the chapter, How To Control Your Cholesterol. This is a dramatic way of seeing how the types of foods and the way they are prepared can change the amount of calories, fat, cholesterol and soluble fiber you eat.

Complete your charts by using the information on the labels of packaged foods and books containing this type of information. See Vital Health Facts listed in back of book.

A review of chart #1:

- 51% of the calories are from fat (169.3 gms. x 9 calories/gram divided by 2962 calories). This is much more than the recommended total daily fat intake of 25% to 35% of total daily calories.
    - Saturated fat is 20% of the total calories, should be below 7%.
    - Polyunsaturated fat is 10%, the highest acceptable level.
    - Monounsaturated fat is 18%, which is within the recommended level of up to 20%.
- 554 mg. of cholesterol is very high compared to the recommended level of less than 200 mg. daily.
- 8.9 grams of soluble fiber is below the suggested amount of 10 to 25 grams daily.

DAILY FOOD DIARY—PRESENT EATING STYLE

Food Eaten	Chart #1 Amount	Calories	Total Fat	Satu-rated Fat	Poly-unsatu-rated Fat	Mono-unsatu-rated Fat	Choles-terol	Soluble Fiber
		Grams	Grams	Grams	Grams	Grams	Milli-Grams	Grams
fried egg	1	95	7	2.7	0.8	2.7	278	0
bacon	3 slices	110	9	3.3	1.1	4.5	16	0
wheat toast	2 slices	140	2	0.8	0.6	0.8	0	0.6
butter	1 tbs	100	11	7.1	0.4	3.3	31	0
orange juice	1 cup	110	tr	tr	tr	tr	0	0.2
bologna	3 slices	270	24	9.2	2.1	11.4	46	0
Amer. cheese	2 slices	105	9	5.6	0.3	2.5	27	0
wheat bread	2 slices	140	2	0.8	0.6	0.8	0	0.6
mayon-naise	1 tbs	100	11	1.7	5.8	3.2	8	0
potato chips	20 ch	210	14	3.6	7.2	2.4	0	0.1
Coke	12 oz	160	0	0	0	0	0	0
pork chop	3 oz	330	26	9.6	3.0	12.1	88	0
baked potato	1	220	tr	0.1	0.1	tr	0	2.0
butter	1 tbs	100	11	7.1	0.4	3.3	31	0
sour cream	3 tbs	75	9	4.8	0.3	2.1	15	0
cooked carrots	½ cup	35	tr	tr	tr	tr	0	1.0
cooked peas	½ cup	62	tr	tr	0.1	tr	0	2.0
butter	1 tsp	33	3.5	2.4	0.1	1.1	10	0
vegetable salad	2 cups	32	tr	tr	0.3	tr	0	0.4
French dressing	2 tbs	130	12.8	3.0	6.8	2.4	4	0
apple pie	1 slice	405	18.0	4.6	4.4	7.4	0	2.0
Totals	xxx	2962	169.3	66.4	34.4	60.0	554	8.9

As a comparison, look at the delicious food and the quantities on chart #2 and compare the totals on chart #1.

As you can see from chart #2:

1. Fat supplies 28% of the calories(68.7 gms x 9 calories / gram divided by 2202 calories), which is within the recommended total fat intake of 25% to 35% of daily calories. The 28% shows a limited fat intake and yet plenty of food was eaten.

   • Saturated fat is 6% of total calories, within the acceptable amount.

   • Polyunsaturated fat is 6.45%, within the acceptable amount.

   • Monounsaturated fat is 13.5%, good amount but could be more if desired, up to 20%.

2. Cholesterol of 106.25 mg. is well below the 200 mg. limit.

3. A soluble fiber intake of 13.4 grams is within the recommended range of 10 - 25 grams though on the low side.

For more detailed information on the amount of fat to eat, see the section in Chapter Four, How To Determine the Amount of Fat to Eat Daily.

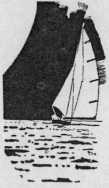

Stay on course.
Fill out your charts.
Use them to set your sail.

DAILY FOOD DIARY—FOR CHOLESTEROL LOWERING

Food Eaten	Amount	Calories	Total Fat	Satu-rated Fat	Poly-unsatu-rated Fat	Mono-unsatu-rated Fat	Choles-terol	Soluble Fiber
(Chart #2)		Grams	Grams	Grams	Grams	Grams	Milli-grams	Grams
orange	1	60	tr	tr	tr	tr	0	0.3
oatmeal	1 cup	145	2.0	0.4	1.0	0.8	0	2.0
1% milk	½ cup	80	1.5	0.75	tr	0.4	3.5	0
wheat toast	1 slice	70	1.0	0.4	0.3	0.4	0	0.3
marga-rine	1 tsp	33	3.5	0.6	1.6	1.3	0	0
apple	1	125	1.0	0.1	0.2	tr	0	1.5
bean soup	2 cups	340	12.0	3.0	3.6	4.4	2.0	2.5
lettuce	1 bowl	20	tr	tr	0.2	tr	0	0.2
olive oil dressing	1 tbs	12.0	14.0	2.0	2.0	10.0	0	0
orange gelatin	1 cup	140	0	0	0	0	0	0
oat bran muffin	1	100	3.5	0.5	1.0	1.9	0	2.0
marga-rine	1 tsp	33	3.5	0.6	1.6	1.3	0	0
almonds	1 oz	167	15.0	1.4	3.1	9.6	0	0
roasted chicken	3 oz	140	3.0	0.9	0.7	1.1	73.0	0
baked potato	1	220	tr	0.1	0.1	tr	0	2.0
low fat plain yo-gurt with chives	2 tbs	24	0.5	0.3	tr	0.1	1.75	0
broccoli	1 cup	45	tr	0.1	0.2	tr	0	2.0
cauli-flower	½ cup	15	tr	tr	tr	tr	0	0.5
parmesan chesse	2 tbs	50	4.0	2.0	tr	0.8	8.0	0
Sherbet	1 cup	270	4.0	2.4	0.1	1.1	14.0	0
Totals	xxx	2202	68.7	15.55	15.7	33.2	106.25	13.4

(tr = trace amount)

YOUR DAILY FOOD DIARY

Food Eaten	Chart #3 Amount	Calories Grams	Total Fat Grams	Satu- rated Fat Grams	Poly- unsatu- rated Fat Grams	Mono- unsatu- rated Fat Grams	Choles- terol Milli- Grams	Soluble Fiber Grams
Totals	xxx							

6

FOOD LOGISTICS

As you have discovered, the food you eat is your first line of defense and attack for controlling your cholesterol. To enable you to have a greater degree of control, you will need to make some minor changes or modifications.

There are four areas of concern:

1. Planning   determine the foods that are best for helping you control your cholesterol level

2. Shopping   use a list of needed foods to help you avoid the foods detrimental to your progress

3. Preparation   use cooking methods best suited to controlling your cholesterol level

4. Eating out   take your time ordering and ask questions about how food is prepared

Major changes in your body chemistry and your overall well-being can be brought about by small changes in your eating habits and lifestyle. The changes in eating habits begin with what you buy and bring home from the grocery store and what you eat when dining out.

PLANNING: WHAT FOODS TO EAT

Review your overall eating pattern and see where you need to make changes to control your cholesterol. Do you need to stop eating fatty foods such as fried foods, lunch meats, hot dogs, hamburgers and other meats and begin eating more fish and nonmeat meals with beans, lentils or tofu?

In planning what foods you should be eating, ask yourself:

- What is the fat content?
    What type of fats (you want low saturated fat content)?
    What percentage of calories per serving come from fat?
- What is the cholesterol content?
- How many calories per serving?
- Does it have any soluble fiber?
- Is it a complex rather than a simple carbohydrate?

If you eat few foods high in saturated fat, an occasional high saturated fat food won't raise your blood cholesterol level. If you anticipate a high saturated fat, high cholesterol day, eat an especially low saturated fat, low cholesterol diet the day before and the day after. For example, if you are planning to attend a picnic or reception, sandwich that day between two days of highly modified eating.

Remember, your goal is to limit the saturated fat and cholesterol in your diet each day. You don't need to cut out all the high saturated fat and high cholesterol foods. But try to substitute one or two low saturated fat or low cholesterol foods each day; soon you will reach your goal of a low saturated fat, low cholesterol diet. This is called behavior modification and should be done in a peaceful and controlled fashion. All behavior modification is best reinforced with objective (without prejudice or emotions) thought and information.

The number and size of servings should be adjusted to reach and maintain your desirable weight. Use the chart below to be sure you are eating an adequate amount from each food category daily.

RECOMMENDED DAILY FOOD PLANNING GUIDE

Food Category	Nutrients	Number of Servings
Dairy products 　1 serving 　　1 cup milk/yogurt 　　1½ oz. cheese 　　½ cup cottage 　　cheese	Protein Fat Carbohydrates	2 for adults 3 for teenagers 3 when pregnant or 　breastfeeding
Eggs 　1 serving 　　2 eggs	Protein Fat	3 yolks/week Unlimited whites
Meats, poultry, Fish 　1 serving 　　2 oz. cooked Meat the size & thickness of woman's palm = 3 to 5 oz., man's = 5 to 7 oz.	Protein Fat	1 to 2 No more than 4 oz. 　3 to 5 days/week
Beans 　1 serving 　　1 cup cooked 　　　dried peas, 　　　beans, lentils, Tofu 　　2 tbs. Natural 　　　peanut butter	Protein Carbohydrates Fat, very little	2 to 4 per week
Fats and oils	Fat	No more than 6 to 　8 teaspoons a day
Fruits 　1 serving 　　½ cup juice 　　½ cup cooked 　　1 cup raw 　　1 medium fresh 　　½ grapefruit 　　wedge of melon 　　½ cup berries 　　¼ cup dried	Carbohydrates	2 to 4
Vegetables 　1 serving 　　½ cup juice 　　½ cup cooked 　　1 cup raw	Carbohydrates	3 to 5

continued on next page

Food Category	Nutrients	Number of Servings
Whole grain products 1 serving 1 slice bread ½ bun or English muffin 1 small roll, biscuit or muffin 4 to 6 crackers ½ cup cooked cereal, rice or pasta 1 oz. ready to eat cereal	Carbohydrates Protein Fat, a little	6 to 11

SHOPPING FOR FOODS

The supermarket is the ideal place to begin making the changes in what you will be eating. Choose a wide variety of foods that are:
- Low fat
- Low-cholesterol
- High soluble fiber

Some basic suggestions for shopping are:

- Never go grocery shopping when you are hungry or near mealtime. This is usually when your willpower is at its lowest and impulse buying is at its highest which leads to buying inappropriate foods.
- Have a shopping list which has only high soluble fiber, low fat and low cholesterol items listed. Buy only those items.
- Head for the produce section first, stocking up on fresh fruits and vegetables.
- Choose low-fat meats, poultry, fish, and dairy products, dried beans and peas, whole grain products, and vegetable oils high in monounsaturated fats.
- Buy mostly from the outside aisles. Commercially prepared foods and many "impulse" items are placed on the inner aisles and are often the sources of hidden fats, especially saturated and hydrogenated fat.

- Read and compare food labels for fat, fiber and cholesterol content.

If you stock your kitchen shelves with foods that are low in saturated fat and cholesterol, it will be much easier to adjust your eating habits. With a little additional thought, time and effort in the beginning you can learn to shop for these foods quickly. Treat yourself with kindness by making these minor adjustments.

Reading and Understanding Food Labels

Nutritional information on packaged food products helps you select foods suitable to your dietary requirements. Nutrition labels identify the types and amounts of nutrients provided in the packaged food. Reading labels will help you find foods that are low in fat, especially saturated fat, and cholesterol.

When shopping, compare labels. You want to buy foods with low total fat and no or low saturated fat and cholesterol. All food labels list the product's ingredients in order by weight. The ingredient in the greatest amount by weight is listed first. The ingredient in the least amount by weight is listed last.

To avoid too much total or saturated fat, limit your use of products that list a fat or oil first or that list many fat and oil ingredients. The list below identifies the names of common saturated fat and cholesterol sources in foods.

SOURCES OF SATURATED FAT AND CHOLESTEROL		
Animal fat	Egg and egg yolk solids	Palm kernel oil
Bacon fat	Ham fat	Palm oil
Beef fat	Hardened fat or oil	Pork fat
Butter	Hydrogenated	Turkey fat
Chicken fat	vegetable oil	Vegetable oil*
Cocoa butter	Lamb fat	Vegetable
Coconut	Lard	shortening
Coconut oil	Meat fat	Whole milk
Cream		solids

* Could be coconut or palm oil

Check the types of fat on the ingredient list of the package and ask yourself some questions, such as:

- Is it an animal fat, coconut oil, palm oil, palm kernel oil or hydrogenated vegetable oil? All are high in saturated fat and are the oils you want to avoid.
- Is it corn, cottonseed, safflower, sunflower or soybean oil? All are high in polyunsaturated fat and may be used in moderate amounts.
- Is it avocado, canola (rapeseed), olive oil? All are high in monounsaturated fat and are the oils you want to use most often.

Most labels show the amount of total fat in grams per serving. The label may also list the:

- Percentage of calories from fat
- Amount of saturated fats
- Amount of polyunsaturated fat
- Amount of monounsaturated fat
- Amount of cholesterol

The amount of monounsaturated fat is not always listed, you can approximate it by doing two steps of basic math:

1. **Add the polyunsaturated and saturated fats**
2. **Subtract them from the total fat content which will give you the amount of monounsaturated fat**

With the information on the label, you can compare the fat and cholesterol content of different products. Choose products with a low proportion of saturated fat and a high proportion of monounsaturated fat.

The following charts show how to identify products with lower saturated fat and cholesterol. These charts help you understand product labels more easily. Labels give the amount of fat in grams (g) and cholesterol in milligrams (mg) per serving.

Take note, 2%, 1% and skim milk have less fat and cholesterol than whole milk. Soft margarine (liquid or tub variety) has less saturated fat and cholesterol than stick butter or margarine.

When comparing nutrition information, be sure you are comparing the same serving size with each item, for example, Tbs. with Tbs., cup with cup, lb. with lb. etc. Notice that some brands of margarine information are in tsp. and other brands are in Tbs.
Following a low saturated fat, low cholesterol diet is a balancing act. It requires eating the variety of foods necessary to supply the nutrients your body needs without eating:

- Too much saturated fat
- Too much cholesterol
- Too many calories

Nutrition Information Per Serving	Whole milk	2% milk	Skim milk
Serving size	1 cup	1 cup	1 cup
Calories	150	121	86
Protein	8 g	8 g	8 g
Carbohydrates	11 g	12 g	12 g
Total fat	8 g	5 g	< 1 g
Polyunsaturated	< 1 g	< 1 g	0 g
Saturated	5 g	3 g	< 1 g
Cholesterol	33 mg	18 mg	4 mg

< means less than   The amount of monounsaturated fat is not listed

Nutrition Information Per Serving	Butter stick	margarine tub
Serving size	1Tb	1Tb
Calories	101	101
Protein	0.1 g	0.1 g
Carbohydrates	0.1 g	0.1 g
Fat(100% calories from fat)	11.4 g	11.4 g
Polyunsaturated	0.4 g	3.9 g
Saturated	7.1 g	1.8 g
Cholesterol	31 mg	0 mg

One way to assure variety, and at the same time a well-balanced diet, is to select foods each day from each of the following food groups. Also select different foods from within groups, especially foods low in saturated fat (second column). Portions and the size of each portion should be adjusted to reach and maintain your desirable weight. As a guide, the recommended daily number of portions is listed for each food group.

MAKING THE RIGHT CHOICE

Food Groups	Choose	Go Easy On	Decrease

Meat
(2 to 3 servings per week, total 6-9 oz.)
	lean cuts of meat with fat trimmed, such as:
	• beef
	  round, sirloin, chuck, loin
	• lamb
	  leg, arm, loin rib
	• pork
	  tenderloin, leg (fresh), shoulder (arm, picnic)
	• veal
	  all trimmed cuts except ground
			"Prime, Choice" Fatty cuts of meat, such as:
			• beef
			  corned beef brisket, regular ground short ribs
			• pork
			  spareribs, blade roll fresh frankfurters sausage, bacon luncheon meats organ meats

Poultry, Fish, & Shellfish (up to 4 oz./day)	poultry without skin fish shellfish canned fish packed in water		goose, domestic duck self-basting turkey caviar, roe
Dairy Products (2 servings/day; 3 servings for teens or when pregnant or breastfeeding)	skim milk, 1% milk, low-fat butter-milk, low-fat evaporated or nonfat milk low-fat or nonfat yogurt low-fat soft cheeses like cottage, pot, farmer, sapsago cheeses labeled 2 to 6 grams fat/oz.	2% milk part-skim ricotta part-skim or imitation hard cheeses "light" cream cheese "light" sour cream	whole milk & its products; cream, half & half, non-dairy creamers, imitation milk products, whipped cream custard style yogurt neufchatel brie, swiss, Amer-ican, mozzarella, feta, cheddar, muenster cream cheese sour cream
Eggs (3 yolks/week)	egg whites		egg yolks

Food Groups	Choose	Go Easy On	Decrease
Fats & Oils (up to 6 to 8 tsp./day)	unsaturated vegetable oils: olive, canola, peanut, safflower, corn, sesame, sunflower, soybean margarine made with unsaturated oils, liquid or tub	nuts seeds avocados olives	butter, coconut oil, palm oil, palm kernel oil, lard, bacon fat margarine or shortening made with saturated fat
Breads, Cereals, Pasta, Rice, Dried Peas and Beans	whole grain bread, English muffins, dinner rolls, pita, rice cakes low-fat crackers; matzo, bread sticks, kavli, rye krisp, saltines, zwieback, soda crackers, pretzels hot cereals, most cold dry cereals pasta; plain noodles, spaghetti, macaroni any grain rice dried peas & beans, split peas, black-eyed peas, chick peas, kidney beans, navy beans, lentils, soybeans, tofu	store-bought pancakes, waffles, biscuits, muffins, cornbread	croissant, butter rolls, sweet rolls, Danish pastry, doughnuts most snack crackers; cheese crackers butter crackers those made with saturated oils granola-type cereals made saturated oils pasta & rice prepared with cream, butter or cheese sauce; egg noodles
Fruits and Vegetables (2 to 4 servings fruit, 3 to 5 servings vegetables/day)	fresh, frozen (plain), canned or dried fruits and vegetables		vegetables prepared in butter, cream or sauce
Sweets and Snacks (avoid too many sweets)	low-fat frozen desserts; sherbet, sorbet, Italian ice, frozen yogurt, popsicles low-fat cakes; angel food cake low-fat cookies; fig bars, gingersnaps low-fat snacks; plain pop-corn, nonfat beverages; carbonated drinks, unsweetened juices, tea	ice milk, homemade cakes, cookies & pies using saturated oils sparingly fruit crisps & cobblers	high-fat frozen desserts, ice cream, frozen tofu high-fat cakes; most store-bought cakes, pound & frosted cakes store-bought; pies, most cookies, candy, high-fat snacks; chips, buttered popcorn high-fat beverages; frappes, milkshakes, floats, eggnog

PREPARATION OF FOODS

When you prepare foods at home, you have a great opportunity to control:

- Selection of foods
- Ingredients
- How foods are prepared

You will be able to regulate your cholesterol levels greatly by making minor changes in the foods you select and how you prepare them.

An aspect of cooking to control your cholesterol is using vegetable oils low in saturated fat and high in mono-unsaturated fat and avoiding oils and fats high in saturated fat. Below is a guide to help you select the more favorable oils.

CHECK YOUR COOKING FATS AND OILS			
Oil	Fat %	Characteristics	Cooking Uses
Almond	Sat. 7% Mono. 64% Poly. 28%	Strong, toated nutty Flavor; low smoke point, Not good for deep frying	Salad dressings, Chicken salad; Small amount in Nutty baked items
Avocado	Sat. 7% Mono. 71% Poly. 29%	Rich; high smoke point	Great in salads; appropriate for fast and deep frying and sauteing
Bacon fat	Sat. 39% Mono. 9% Poly. 12%	Low smoke point	Frying
Butter	Sat. 66% Mono. 30% Poly. 4%	Low smoke point	Used in baking
Canola (Rapeseed)	Sat. 6% Mono. 60% Poly. 3%	Light, clear, bland; high smoke point; all purpose	Very good for baking; blends well for salad dressings
Chicken fat	Sat. 31% Mono. 47% Poly. 22%		Frying

continued on next page

Oil	Fat %	Characteristics	Cooking Uses
Coconut	Sat. 90% Mono. 6% Poly. 2%		Used in many commercially baked goods
Corn	Sat. 13% Mono. 24% Poly. 59%	Good, "corny" taste; general purposes	Good for baking, great for pie crust and making popcorn
Lard	Sat. 41% Mono. 47% Poly. 12%	Not much flavor	Used in baking and frying
Margarine	Fats not broken down because individual margarines vary greatly and there is no "average" margarine. When selecting a margarine choose one with an acceptable liquid vegetable oil listed first on the ingredient list and with the lowest level of saturated fat.		
Olive	Sat. 14% Mono. 77% Poly. 8%	Extra Virgin: Fruity, robust flavor; deep greenish-gold; point medium smoke	Perfect in salads stews, sauces & cheese dishes good for light sautéing
		Classico: Subtle, traditional flavor; medium-high smoke point	For meat, poultry vegetables, sauces & salads; perfect for pan-frying
		Extra Light: Very slight mild flavor and light bouquet; light gold color high smoke point	Suitable for all kinds of cooking, from sauteing delicate fish to baking cakes & muffins; ideal for shallow & deep frying
Palm	Sat. 50% Mono. 38% Poly. 10%		Used in many commercially baked items
Palm Kernel	Sat. 85% Mono. 12% Poly. 32%		Used mostly in commercially baked items
Peanut	Sat. 17% Mono. 46% Poly. 32%	Slightly heavy, nutty flavor; can "flash" at high temperatures	Perfect for stir-fries; good for salads

continued on next page

Oil	Fat %	Characteristics	Cooking Uses
Safflower	Sat. 9% Mono. 12% Poly. 75%	Bland; general use	All types of cooking; use to dilute strong flavored oils; blends well
Sesame	Sat. 14% Mono. 40% Poly. 42%	Made from untoasted seeds is light & bland flavor; from toasted seeds is rich with strong flavor	Untoasted for stir-fries, salads & pan frying Toasted in small quantities for salad dressings and Oriental dishes
Solid vegetable shortening	Sat. 32% Mono. 53% Poly. 15%	High smoke point	Used in baking and deep frying
Soy	Sat. 14% Mono. 23% Poly. 58%	Prominent taste if unrefined; high smoke point	General use
Sunflower	Sat. 10% Mono. 20% Poly. 66%	Almost tasteless and odorless; all purpose	Good for salads, stir-fries, frying & sauteing; blends well; may be used to dilute stronger oils
Walnut	Sat. 9% Mono. 23% Poly. 63%	Rich, slightly nutty low smoke point	Excellent for salad dressing; sautéing on low heat; toss with pasta or in potato or chicken salad

Note: The fat composition of the above oils can vary depending on the source.

In case you have not noticed from the above chart, CHECK YOUR COOKING FATS AND OILS, be sure to take a look at the saturated fat content of:

- Coconut oil
- Palm oil
- Palm kernel oil

This should give you a clear idea why certain commercial foods must be avoided. Read labels!

A quick glance at LINING UP THE PREFERABLE OILS chart below, reveals that:

- Both Almond and Avocado oils have the best combination for being low in saturated fat and high in monounsaturated. Unfortunately these oils are not general purpose oils and are not readily available.
- Canola oil is the next best choice. It is the lowest in saturated fat and high in monounsaturated fat, is an all purpose oil, and is readily available in stores.
- Olive oil is the highest in monounsaturated fat but has more saturated fat than the other three. Olive oil is a good choice, is versatile, and readily available.

LINING UP THE PREFERABLE OILS

Saturated Fat		*Monounsaturated Fat*	
Canola	6%	Olive	77%
Almond	7%	Avocado	71%
Avocado	7%	Almond	64%
Safflower	9%	Canola	60%
Sunflower	10%	Peanut	46%
Corn	13%	Sesame	40%
Olive	14%	Corn	24%

Put bottles of various types of vegetable oils in your freezer overnight. In the morning those low in saturated fat will pour freely, but those higher in saturated fat will be less pourable. Try it and see!

Low Fat Cooking Tips

Vegetables
- Steam, boil or bake; saute or stir-fry in small amount of broth or water instead of oil or butter.

- Season with herbs, spices, lime or lemon juice rather than with sauces, butter or margarine.
- Use lemon juice or vinegar with water and herbs for salad dressing.
- When sauteing meats, drain all excess fat before continuing with cooking.
- Bake poultry stuffing separately rather than inside poultry.

Meat, fish and poultry

- Remove skin from poultry before cooking.
- Trim fat from meat before and after cooking.
- Roast, bake, broil, or simmer.
- Cook on rack so fat will drain off.
- Baste with fat-free ingredients such as wine, tomato juice or lemon juice instead of fatty drippings. If you feel you must baste with a fat, use a monounsaturated vegetable oil.
- Use nonstick pan for cooking so that added fat will not be necessary.
- Heat slowly so that meat will brown in its own juices, eliminating the need for butter or oil.
- Chill broths and soups until fat becomes solid on top, easily removed and disposed of.

Baked goods

- Try whole grain flours to enhance flavors when using fewer fat and cholesterol containing ingredients.
- Try using oat bran, rice bran and rolled oats for baked items.
- Use monounsatured oils in place of melted or solid shortenings, butter and margarine.
- Use low fat, nonfat milk or fruit juice when whole milk called for in recipe.
- Use 2 egg whites in place of each whole egg called for.
- In cookie, cake and muffins recipes, replace one half of vegetable oil with applesauce.

Miscellaneous

- Prepare soups, stews and gravies ahead of time and refrigerate till able to skim fat off top. To hurry the process, place in freezer for short time or place large jar of ice cubes in soup, stew or gravy. Or use large fat skimmer to pour off fat and avoid the cooling process.
- Limit egg yolks to one per serving when making egg dishes and use additional egg whites for bulking out the serving.
- Use nonstick spray made from vegetable oil or use nonstick pans that require no greasing. If you have neither, put a couple drops of vegetable oil in pan, spread it around and then lightly wipe out with paper towel.
- Eat at least one or two meatless meals per week, including beans, soup, tofu, or lentils.
- Eat fish or seafood two to three times per week.

Lowfat dessert ideas:
- Fresh fruit
- Angel food cake
- Sherbet
- Gelatin
- Ice milk/light ice cream
- Frozen low fat yogurt
- Sorbet

Lowfat snacks
- Air popped popcorn seasoned with spices--onion, garlic, etc.
- Plain nonfat yogurt with chopped fresh fruit added.
- Raw vegetables--carrots, snow peas, cauliflower, broccoli, green beans.
- Fresh fruit.
- Toasted shredded wheat squares sprinkled with small amount of grated parmesan cheese.
- Toasted whole grain English muffin or whole grain bread with small amount nonsugar jelly.
- Toasted plain corn tortillas.
- Rye krisp, soda crackers, melba toast.
- Beverages--water, skim milk, fruit or vegetable juice, mineral water with a twist of lemon or lime.

SUBSTITUTIONS	
Instead of	Use
Sour cream	Plain low-fat yogurt or blended or whipped low-fat cottage cheese
Mayonnaise	Mustard for sandwiches or Yogurt mixed with mustard, lemon juice, herbs and spices
Cream	Evaporated skim milk
Whole milk	1%, nonfat or skim milk
1 Tbs. butter	1 Tbs. soft margarine or ¾ Tbs. vegetable oil
Butter on vegetables	Sprinkle on Butter Buds or Molly McButter
Pouring melted fat over	Use pastry brush to put on fat--much less used
Greasing pans with shortening	Vegetable cooking spray use nonstick pans
Whole milk cheese	1% cottage cheese, low-fat American cheese, farmer/pot cheese, partskim mozzarella, combine parmesan and sapsago for spaghetti
Solid shortenings	Soft margarine with acceptable liquid oil listed first or just use vegetable oil, ie. canola oil
Melted butter or margarine	Olive or canola oil
Ground beef	Low-fat ground veal or turkey/chicken breast
Barbecued ribs	Chicken barbecued without skin
Meats	Tofu
Lunch meats	Sliced turkey, chicken or lean roast beef, water packed tuna fish

Instead of	Use
Commercial soups may be high in fat	Homemade bean, split pea, vegetable or minestrone soup
Chocolate	3 Tbs. cocoa plus 1 Tbs. mono-unsaturated oil for each square (1 oz.) of chocolate
Peanut butter with hydrogenated oil	Natural peanut butter with no hydrogenated oil; store jar upside down

EATING OUT

Eating out has become a national pastime. Foods in restaurants can be a prime source of hidden fats. Too often an individual on a cholesterol controlling diet overreacts to the need of being careful when eating out. The classic comment is, "I won't be able to go out to eat anymore." Nothing could be further from the truth. However, you will have to follow some definite guidelines. Since adjustment is the height of personal intelligence, be intelligent, make the adjustment.

Eating anywhere (restaurants, friends' homes, picnics, hospital, air and train travel) other than at home does require some additional effort on your part. But it doesn't have to be a traumatic event, and you shouldn't become a recluse just because you need to be watchful of what you eat. By keeping a few facts in mind you can enjoy eating out no matter what the setting.

Some ideas to help you when eating out:

- Choose the restaurant carefully by calling the restaurant in advance and asking the following questions:

  - Is there a salad bar?
  - How are the meat, chicken and fish dishes prepared?

- Are there low fat and high fiber selections on the menu?
- Can you have menu items broiled or baked without added fat instead of fried?

The more frequently you eat out, the more important these issues can become. Seafood restaurants usually offer broiled, baked or poached fish, and you can often request butter and sauces on the side so you can control the amount you eat. Many steak houses offer small steaks and have salad bars.

- Try ethnic cuisines. Italian and Asian restaurants often feature low fat dishes. You must be selective and alert to portion size. Try a small serving of pasta or fish in a tomato sauce at an Italian restaurant. Many Chinese, Japanese, and Thai dishes include plenty of steamed vegetables and a high proportion of vegetables to meat. Steamed rice, steamed noodle dishes and vegetarian dishes are good choices too. Some Latin American restaurants feature a variety of fish and chicken dishes low in fat.

- Make sure you get what you want; don't be intimidated by the atmosphere, menu, waiter, friends, or anything else. Here are just a few things you can do to make sure you are in control of the situation when you eat out:

  - Ask how various foods are prepared.
  - Select clear rather than cream soups.
  - Do not hesitate to request that one food be substituted for another.
  - Order appetizers low in cholesterol and/or saturated fat such as seafood cocktail or fruit or vegetable juice.
  - For main course order pasta with steamed vegetables or tomato sauce.
  - Select a green salad or baked potato in place of french fries.

- Request sauces and salad dressings on the side and use only a small amount.
- Ask that butter not be sent to the table with your rolls or ask for soft margarine.
- Request fruit, sherbet, sorbet or angel food cake for dessert instead of baked goods or frozen desserts which are usually made with ingredients high in saturated fat and cholesterol.
- If you're not very hungry, order two low fat appetizers rather than an entire meal, split a menu item with a friend, get a doggie bag to take half of your meal home, or order a half size portion.
- When you have finished eating, have the waiter clear the dishes away so that you can avoid postmeal nibbling.

- Learn and look for terms on the menu that denote low fat preparation or saturated fat and cholesterol preparation.

  - Terms usually associated with low fat and low cholesterol preparation:

    Steamed
    In its own juice
    Broiled
    Roasted
    Poached
    Dry broiled

  - Terms usually associated with saturated fat and cholesterol preparation:

    Buttery, buttered, in butter sauce
    Sauteed, fried, panfried, crispy, braised
    Creamed, in cream sauce, in its own gravy,
      hollandaise
    Au gratin, parmesan, in cheese sauce, escalloped
    Marinated, stewed, basted
    Casserole, prime, hash, pot pie

If Invited

If you casually inform your friends that you are on a low cholesterol, low fat diet, then they will know how to adjust when they invite you to dinner. If foods are served that are on your no-no list, just take a very small portion and go heavy on the permitted foods. Don't make a big ado and say you aren't allowed to eat something that was served. Remember the principle, the height of intelligence is adjustment.

If you are asked what foods you do not eat, mention such foods as red meat and fried foods. Most people can adjust their menu planning around your food needs if they are interested.

·Don't make eating the center of your life. Eat to live, don't live to eat. Socializing should be the important event rather than the food and drink. Don't be conspicuous or make an issue about what you do or do not eat. Your friends, relatives and everyone else simply do not want to hear it, so keep it to yourself, it's your body chemistry you are taking care of.

Also be aware of pressure to eat foods you shouldn't. Just say, "No thank you," and don't make any explanation. If you do have to take it, just don't eat it. Become a smart politician, stay in control of the situation.

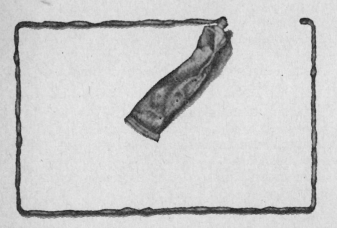

Heather Flint

7

CHOLESTEROL CONCERNS FOR CHILDREN AND ADOLESCENTS

It was believed that most children were at little risk for developing high cholesterol levels and other risk factors for heart diseases affecting the coronary arteries and blood vessels. There may be a family history of cholesterol problems and premature coronary heart disease (CHD). This alone may place your child at a higher risk for developing CHD prematurely in life. However, over the past ten years children are becoming more at risk because of one or more of the following:

- sedentary lifestyles - video games, TV and internet in place of vigorous physical activities
- high-fat and sugar junk food
- overweight or obesity

There is compelling evidence that adult cardiovascular disease (CVD) has it roots in childhood. The atherosclerotic process can begin in childhood and progress slowly into adulthood, when it frequently leads to coronary heart disease (CHD).

Children and adolescents with elevated blood cholesterol, particularly Low Density Lipoprotein (LDL cholesterol) levels, frequently come from families in which there is a high incidence of CHD among adult members. High blood cholesterol occurs in families as a result of both shared environments and genetic factors. Children and adolescents with high cholesterol levels are more likely than the general population to have high levels as adults.

The information in this chapter should be used in conjunction with your child's physician and the rest of the book but most particularly with the chapter, How to Control Your Cholesterol.

WHO SHOULD BE TESTED?

Your children over 2 years of age should be tested if either biological parent has or has had a high cholesterol (above 240) or there is a biological family history of early cardiovascular disease. Family history includes:

- parent, sibling, grandparent, aunt or uncle who experienced one of the following before age 55:

  - myocardial infarction (heart attack)
  - angina pectoris (chest pain due to coronary atherosclerosis)
  - peripheral artery disease
  - cerebrovascular disease (stroke)
  - sudden cardiac death

If none of the above pertain, your child or adolescent should be tested if any of the following pertain to him/her:

- smoking
- diabetes
- obesity (30% or more overweight)
- high blood pressure
- oral contraceptive use

HOW TO BE TESTED

There are a couple of approaches for testing.

1. Nonfasting total blood cholesterol level - this test is done if a parent has high blood cholesterol or other risk factors. See risk factors in the chapter, How Serious Is High Cholesterol.

   • If the results are acceptable (total cholesterol below 170) , then there is nothing to be done except continue with a healthy diet and have the child tested again in 5 years.

   • If the total cholesterol is above 170, then a fasting total lipid profile is done. Fasting is nothing to eat or drink, except water, for 9 - 12 hours before the testing.

   Note: In our opinion, why not just have the fasting total lipid profile done in the beginning? Then there would be no need for a second test if the total cholesterol is above 170. What child, or adult for that matter, enjoys having blood drawn more often than necessary? Get the total picture in the beginning and avoid a second needle stick. The exception to this idea is if it is too difficult to get an early morning appointment which is the only appropriate time for fasting blood work .

2. Fasting total lipid profile (includes total cholesterol, HDL & LDL cholesterol and triglycerides) - done if there is a biological family (parents, siblings, grandparents) history of early cardiovascular disease.

If your child or adolescent has an elevated cholesterol and/or triglyceride level, the findings could be secondary in part to such factors as follows, which should be considered and tested for:

   • obesity
   • pediatric medical conditions such as:
     hypothyroidism (underactive thyroid)
     diabetes

nephrotic syndrome (excessive protein lost in urine)
severe kidney disease
hepatitis/liver disease
auto-immune diseases (conditions where the body makes antibodies against its own organs such as lupus erythematosus)
storage diseases - glycogen storage disease, Tay Sachs disease, Niemann-Pick disease - these are very rare

- teenage conditions such as:
  eating disorders (food avoidance or binging)
  excessive alcohol intake

- medications
  oral contraceptives - "The pill"
  Accutane (an acne medication)
  thiazide diuretics
  steroids/hormones
  epilepsy or seizure medications

CHOLESTEROL LEVELS

For the first few months after a baby is born, most of the change in cholesterol levels is due to an increase of LDL cholesterol. This LDL rise levels off at about two years of age. Over the following years there will be little change in the total cholesterol (150 - 165) and LDL cholesterol (100 or a little lower) levels until the late teens.

HDL cholesterol (55) level is similar in both males and females in the early years but decrease in males when they reach about 15 years of age.

Triglycerides rise at first , then should decrease to about 50 - 60 and rise again to 75 or more by age 20 .

Children with high cholesterol levels tend to have higher levels as adults; children with low cholesterol levels tend to have lower levels as adults. This is not an exact assessment however, because lifestyles can change particularly diet and physical activity.

Cholesterol Levels Between 2 and 19 Years of Age		
Category	Total Cholesterol	LDL
Acceptable	less than 170	less than 110
Borderline	170 - 199	110 - 129
High	200 or above	130 or above

Triglycerides levels		
Age	above 2, below 10	10, below 20
Acceptable	less than 75	less than 85
Borderline	75 - 99	85 - 129
High	100 or above	130 or above

Obesity is a major cause of mild increases in triglycerides.

> **It is important that your child or adolescent understands that high cholesterol is not a disease, but a major risk factor for atherosclerosis.**

WHAT TO DO IF CHOLESTEROL LEVELS ARE HIGH

There are three aspects to consider in helping to control your child's or adolescent's cholesterol levels:

1. Changing the kinds and amounts of foods eaten is the primary approach to controlling cholesterol levels. The goal is to reduce the LDL cholesterol level.

   • For LDL cholesterol level between 110 - 129:

   lower it to below 110

- For LDL cholesterol level 130 or more:

    lower it to below 130 as a minimal goal

    lower it to below 110 as an ideal goal which is also preferred for risk reduction.

2. Increase in physical activity/weight loss is the second aspect of lowering elevated cholesterol levels.

3. Medication

Change the Foods

It would be very beneficial to your child or adolescent if the all family members above age two were to follow the dietary recommendations below. This is a healthy way of eating for those over two years of age and the child or adolescent would not feel different or deprived.

It is important that the foods provide adequate energy and nutrients for growth and to maintain appropriate weight. A wide variety of foods should be eaten to assure a sufficient intake of protein, carbohydrates and fat along with other essentials such as calcium, iron and other minerals and vitamins. To this end, it may be advantageous to seek the assistance of a qualified nutritionist or a registered dietician.

Children under two years of age should not follow this program because they need a relatively high calorie intake to maintain their rapid growth. Since fat is high in calories, children under two need to get more than 30% of their calories from fat to get all the calories they need to ensure their normal growth.

Changes:

- Eat less fat - 30% or less of total daily calorie intake

    saturated fat - less than 10% of total daily calories

    polyunsaturated fat - up to 10% of total calories

    monounsaturated fat - approximately 10% of total calories

- Eat less cholesterol - 100 mg per 1000 calories, not to exceed 300 mg per day

- Eat more complex carbohydrates - vegetables, fruits, and whole grains

For a more in-depth explanation, see the chapter, How to Control Your Cholesterol.

After your child has followed the dietary changes for three to six months, his/her cholesterol levels should be rechecked to see if the LDL goal has been met. If the LDL goal has been met, then the program should be carefully intensified somewhat and the cholesterol levels checked yearly.

If the LDL goal has not been met, the following additional dietary modifications may be suggested by your physician:

- Eat less fat - 25% or less (no less than 20%) of total daily calorie intake

- Eat less saturated fat - less than 7% of total daily calorie intake

- Eat less cholesterol - 75 mg per 1000 calories, not to exceed 200 mg per day

Eat less fat

Some of the easiest ways to eat less fat, especially saturated fat is to substitute:

Instead of	Have
french fries	1/2 serving or baked potato
home fries	mashed potatoes
fried eggs	scrambled egg whites with 1 yolk
fried chicken/fish	baked or broiled
fried hamburgers	grilled
hot dogs	turkey/chicken hot dogs

grilled cheese sandwich	grilled cheese on whole grain bread with low fat cheese and soft veg oil spread
cheese hamburger	ground lean round, turkey breast or veggie burger
potato chips	soy based chips or air-popped corn
pizza	one or two slices of low fat cheese pizza with vegetable topping, infrequently
white bread & rolls	whole grain breads and rolls
regular milk shake	milk shake of 1% milk and light ice cream
regular ice cream	light ice cream, low fat frozen yogurt, sherbet, sorbet, fruit popsicles
whole milk	1% or skim milk
sour cream	low fat yogurt
tuna packed in oil	tuna packed in water
regular salad dressings	low fat salad dressings
regular peanut butter	natural or low fat peanut butter
butter	soft tub margarines made with liquid canola, saflower, sunflower or, corn oils
regular yogurt	low fat yogurt
regular granola	low fat granola or other low fat cereal such as: corn flakes, cheerios, a bran cereal, oatmeal, etc.
regular cheese	low fat cheese
regular lunch meats	low fat lunch meats or slices of homemade roast chicken, turkey or beef
commercial cookies, cakes, pies, puddings	home made cookies, cakes, pies, puddings made with acceptable ingredients

Making your own desserts and muffins can be very beneficial in helping in your child eating less fat, especially saturated fat. You can:

- use a high monounsaturated fat and low saturated fat oil such as canola oil or olive oil for the vegetable oil or shortening in a recipe.

- replace at least half or more of the vegetable oil with applesauce.

- use canola oil when making pie crust rather than a hard or soft shortening.

To calculate how many calories from fat your child may eat, you can do the following:

1. From the chart below, determine how many total calories may be eaten daily. For example let's use 2180 calories for a 13 year old girl.

RECOMMENDED DAILY CALORIC INTAKE FOR CHILDREN AND ADOLESCENTS		
Calories to maintain weight		
Age (years)	Girls	Boys
2	1,160	1,250
3	1,270	1,530
4	1,430	1,520
5	1,550	1,680
6	1,760	1,840
7	1,530	1,590
8	1,720	1,750
9	2,000	1,970
10	2,260	2,230
11	1,730	1,930
12	1,950	2,180
13	2,180	2,430
14	2,350	2,780
15	2,130	2,540
16	2,240	2,780
17	2,250	2,970
18	2,250	3,130

Source: National Research Council

Eating the recommended amount of calories to maintain a normal weight will help those who need to lose weight.

2. Since 30% of the calories may come from total fat, you determine what 30% is by multiplying the total calories times 30%. That would be:

    2180 x .30 = 654 calories may come from fat.

    Many packaged food labels list how many calories come from fat per serving which can be very helpful. Sometimes only grams, not calories, are listed so it is helpful to be able to determine how many grams of fat may be eaten daily.

    Since there are 9 calories per gram of fat, you divide the calories of fat by 9. That would be:

    654 ÷ 9 = 72.6 grams of fat may be eaten daily.

3. Since no more than 10% of total calories may come from saturated fat, you determine 10% by multilying the total calories times 10%. That would be:

    2180 x .10 = 218 calories can come from saturated fat. This means, of the total 654 fat calories, 218 can come from saturated fat.

    For how many grams of saturated fat are permitted, divide the 218 by 9 which is:

    218 ÷ 9 = 24 grams of saturated fat. This means that of the total 72.6 grams of fat, 24 of them may come from saturated fat.

If your child or adolescent is overweight, eating less fat will help him/her to lose weight. If he/she is not overweight, then you must be sure that sufficient carbohydrates and protein are eaten to replace the calories lost from eating less fat.

Eat less cholesterol

Even though saturated fat raises blood cholesterol levels more than cholesterol, it is also important to decrease the amount of cholesterol eaten.

Cholesterol is found only in animal products such as:
- egg yolk
- dairy products
- meats, fish, poultry

See cholesterol content of some common foods in the chapter, How to Control Your Cholesterol.

To decrease the amount of cholesterol your child or adolescent eats, try:

- Using 2 egg whites for every egg called for in a recipe or at least decrease the number and/or size of yolks used.

- Have some meatless meals a couple times a week by using beans, lentils, pasta or tofu in place of meat. See the cookbook section for recipe suggestions.

Remember, there is no cholesterol in:

fruits	grains
vegetables	nuts
legumes	seeds

Eat more complex carbohydrates

Complex carbohydrates which are comprised mainly of starch and some sugar are vegetables, whole grains, legumes, nuts and seeds. Fruits are simple carbohydrates comprised of mostly sugars and some starch. The less refined the carbohydrates the better.

As we all know, it is sometimes difficult to get children and adolescents to eat a wide variety of vegetables. But vegetables are important for a well balanced food intake and especially when trying to control cholesterol levels.

These are the foods that can be used to replace the foods that are high in fat.

Since using cream and cheese sauces on vegetables is not recommended in this program, you may need to be creative with herbs and spices to make vegetables appetizing. Of course once in awhile you could make a low fat cream, yogurt or cheese sauce.

Raw vegetables such as carrots, celery, broccoli, cauliflower served with a low fat dip or salsa may be more acceptable than cooked vegetables.

For a product to be a whole grain product, it must have the "whole grain" listed first on the ingredient list. The word "whole" must be included. For example, whole wheat bread must have "whole wheat", not wheat flour, as the first ingredient. When selecting cereals look for whole grains as the first ingredient - whole rolled oat, whole oats, whole corn, etc.

Try including beans, lentils and rice in more meals. See cookbook section for recipe ideas.

Have nuts, seeds and raisins or other dried fruit mixture available for snacks. Just keep these to a minimum because of the high natural sugar content of dried fruit and fat content of the nuts and seeds. Have fresh fruit and cut up raw vegetables available for snacks.

It's a good idea to read the section on carbohydrates in the chapter, How to Control Your Cholesterol.

Increase Physical Activity

Today many of our children and adolescents have become much less physically active than in decades past. This is due in large part to the sedentary activities of television, video games, passive entertainment and internet use.

If this applies to your children, do your best to limit TV, computer and video game time. Encourage your children to become more physically active and interact with them.

Children learn by watching adults. If you are physically active, there is a better chance your children will be also.

Get the whole family involved in physical activity. Some suggestions are:

- Take daily walks after dinner.

- Plan hikes or biking together - in neighbor-hood, parks, mountains, beach, bike paths.

- Play games together - volley ball, tennis, ping. pong, croquet, golf (carry clubs), shooting basketballs, swimming, etc.

- Jumping rope, skating.

- Walking or carefully riding a bike to the store, school or friend's house rather than driving or being driven in a car.

- Using stairs rather than elevator or escalator.

- Park car a distance from store or other destination to increase walking when doable.

Most of the above ideas children can do by themselves or with other children. Joining school or community athletic programs is another option.

Another dimension is helping with activities around the home such as:

cleaning	mowing the lawn	garden work
painting	home repairs	raking leaves

The above are not only healthy physical activities but increase family bonding as well.

If your child or adolescent is overweight, weight loss should occur by increasing physical activity and decreasing the amount of calories eaten.

Medication

Medication is usually only considered for children ten years or older who have not reached their LDL cholesterol goal after six months to one year of following their diet program. This is often the case with hereditary disorders of high cholesterol. Medication should only be considered and prescribed by qualified physicians who are experienced in treating these conditions. If medication is ordered, the diet program is still followed.

The minimum goal of medication is to attain an LDL cholesterol level of less than 130. If possible, the level should be brought nearer to 110 or lower. Evidence increasingly shows, the lower, the better.

Medication is considered for those ten years and above whose:

- LDL cholesterol is 190 or higher

- LDL cholesterol is 160 or higher and:

    * there is a positive family history of premature cardio-vascular disease before the age of 55

        or
    * two or more other cardiovascular risk factors are present in the child or adolescent after vigorous attempts have been made to control the following risk factors:

| cigarette smoking | diabetes | physical inactivity |
| high blood pressure | obesity | HDL below 50 |

Type of medications

Implementation requires sound judgement on the part of the physician and clear understanding on the part of the child patient and parents of the side effects and risks of medication as well as the potential benefits.

Medications currently in use to treat children over 10 years of age are the bile acid sequestrants:

- cholestyramine   • colestipol

These medications should not be used if the triglyceride level is over 300 because they may cause the triglycerides to go even higher.   Also these medications have some bothersome side effects.

Something To Remember

When trying to coordinate good health ideas and lifestyle with your child or adolescent, it's best to avoid a dictatorial role and strive for a consultant's or coach's type of role.   Allow your child or adolescent to develop and grow his/her own ideas and insights when working with you and the physician. Encourage your child/adolescent to be part of the planning and decision making.   Help him/her to understand it is never too early to start a heart-healthy lifestyle. Remember what Socrates said, "Knowledge will bring you joy."   What better thought for both you and your child!

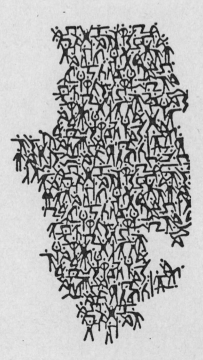

8
QUESTIONS AND ANSWERS

Q. How does the body get cholesterol?
A. Two ways:
    1. Body makes what it needs
    2. From foods of animal origin that we eat

Q. Why should I be concerned about my cholesterol level?
A. Over time, cholesterol, fat and other substances can build up in the walls of your arteries (atherosclerosis) and slow or block the flow of blood to your organs, particularly to your brain, heart, kidneys and lower extremities. This can lead to heart attack, stroke or other cardiovascular conditions. Therefore, the cholesterol level in the bloodstream should be properly regulated.

Q. What are the statistics concerning Americans that give rise to the alarm of cholesterol in relation to cardiovascular disease?
A. The facts are that each year:
    • $1\,{}^{1}/_{2}$ million Americans suffer heart attacks
    • Over ${}^{1}/_{2}$ million suffer their first stroke
Approximately one in two Americans will eventually die from cardiovascular disease. Medical research has established that a high blood cholesterol level is a significant contributor to cardiovascular disease.

Q. What is atherosclerosis?
A. It is a slowly developing process in which the lining of the arteries becomes coated with fatty substances such as

cholesterol. These deposits result in scarring and narrowing of the arteries which eventually may close off completely, either because the deposits have grown together or because a blood clot has caught on the deposits (plaque).

Q. What can be the result of decreased blood flow or blockage of blood flow to organs?

A. a) If in or to your heart, you may have a heart attack
   b) If in or to your brain, you may have a stroke
   c) If in a lower extremity, you may have leg or foot pain, leg or foot ulcers which could even result in gangrene, and possibly lose of limb.

Q. At what age should a person be concerned about cholesterol?

A. Although the problems resulting from high cholesterol do not usually show up until the adult years, the accumulation of fatty substances may begin in childhood. Therefore, forming correct eating and exercising habits in childhood may prevent cholesterol problems later. It is suggested that everyone 20 years of age and older be tested for cholesterol problems. If there is a family history of cholesterol problems or cardio-vascular disease , then young children, after the age of two, should be tested. If any of the following pertain to your child or adolescent he/she should be tested: obesity, diabetes, high blood pressure, smoking or use of oral contraceptives.

Special Attention
See chapter, Cholesterol Concerns
of Children and Adolescents

Q. What is the first thing I should do if I am concerned about my cholesterol?

A. The first thing you should do is to stop eating foods that contain saturated fat. The next things to do are:

- Read the chapter How To Determine If You Have A Cholesterol Problem
- Ask your doctor to order a total lipid profile blood test
- Read the chapter How to Control Your Cholesterol

Q. Is there more than one test for determining my blood cholesterol level?

A. Yes, there are two separate tests:

    1. The total cholesterol test   2. The total lipid profile

We believe it is important to get the total lipid profile rather than just the total cholesterol. For more information, see the chapter, How To Determine If You Have A Cholesterol Problem.

Q. What will correcting my blood cholesterol levels do?

A. Correcting your cholesterol levels will slow, possibly stop, and perhaps reverse fatty buildup in the walls of the arteries. The process will reduce your risk for cardiovascular problems and may save your life too!!

Q. Is there evidence that lowering my blood cholesterol will help me?

A. Most assuredly yes! The scientific information has been well established that lowering your cholesterol will help ward off cardiovascular disease. It is generally agreed that lowering your cholesterol 1% reduces your risk for heart disease by 2%.

Q. What factors influence my cholesterol level?

A. • Foods you eat   • Stress   • Genetics-family history
    • Weight   • Smoking • Gender
    • Age   • Physical activity/exercise

For a more detailed explanation, see the chapter, Understanding Cholesterol

Q. What is more important to eat less of, saturated fat or cholesterol?

A. The saturated fat that you eat causes blood cholesterol to rise more than the cholesterol you eat. Therefore, it seems to be more important to eat less saturated fat than cholesterol even though you should also decrease the amount of cholesterol you eat.

Q. How do I know what foods are high in saturated fats?

A. Animal products as a group are the major source of saturated fat plus coconut oil, palm kernel oil, palm oil and cocoa butter which are found in many commercially baked goods. Read food labels for ingredients listed and refer to a book containing this type of information. See list of books on last page.

Q. Since olive oil is good for you, may I use it in unlimited quantities?

A. First and foremost, olive oil is a fat and should be used sparingly. However, olive oil is low in saturated fat and high in monounsaturated fat like canola oil and is therefore healthier than some other vegetable oils.

Q. What are the most concentrated sources of saturated fat?

A. • Coconut oil, palm kernel and palm oil are the most concentrated sources of saturated fat. They are from 50 to 90% saturated.
   • Butter is 66% saturated   • Lard is 41% saturated

Q. Which food listed is highest in cholesterol?
   • Peach pie   • Coconut oil   • Cashews
   • Crab meat   • Avocados

A. Of the five foods listed, only crab has cholesterol. Cholesterol is found only in foods of animal origin. It is not in fruits, vegetables or vegetable oils.

Q. Do you reduce the cholesterol content of a piece of beef when you trim the fat?

A. Yes! There is 20% more cholesterol in the fat of cooked beef than in an equal weight of muscle.

Q. What does saturated, monounsaturated and polyunsaturated mean when referring to fats?

A. These three terms have to do with the chemical structure of fatty acids. Fatty acids are composed of chains of carbon atoms that have sites for the attachment of hydrogen atoms. If these sites do not have all the hydrogen atoms they can hold, there is a double bond at that site.

   Saturated - all the sites are filled with hydrogen atoms

   Monounsaturated - there is only *one* double bond

   Polyunsaturated - there are *two or more* double bonds

Q. What are hydrogenated fats?
A. These are unsaturated fats (oils) that have been changed from their natural liquid state to a solid state by the addition of hydrogen atoms. They are most commonly found in such products as margarines, solid shortenings and commercially baked products. Hydrogenated fats are what make up the trans fatty acids which are as harmful as saturated fats.

Q. Which of the following foods has the highest fat content?
• chocolate ice cream bar   • 10 English walnuts
• 2 $1/2$ oz. lean pork chop
A. Gotcha! The walnuts have the highest at 32 grams of fat. The pork chop has 8 grams while the ice cream has 19 grams. However, even though the walnuts are high in fat they have the most monounsaturated fat which is the good fat.

Q. What foods are high in cholesterol?
A. Cholesterol is found in egg yolks, dairy products, meat, poultry, fish and shellfish. Egg yolks and organ meats (liver, kidney, sweetbread, brain) are particularly rich sources of cholesterol. Fish generally has less cholesterol than meat and poultry. Shellfish vary in cholesterol content but generally also have less cholesterol than meat and poultry.

Q. Which foods listed help lower your cholesterol?
• Liver   • Lentil soup   • Whole wheat bread
• Apples   • Oat bran cereal
A. The soluble fiber helps to lower your cholesterol. Of the foods listed, oat bran, lentils and apples all contain soluble fiber.

Q. What are the "good" HDLs and the "bad" LDLs ?
A. Some cholesterol travels through the bloodstream in high density lipoproteins (HDLs). The HDLs carry cholesterol back to the liver for processing or removal from the body thereby preventing the accumulation of cholesterol in the artery walls. Hence the name, the "good" HDL cholesterol.

Cholesterol traveling in low density lipoproteins (LDLs) is transported from the liver to other parts of the body where it can be used. LDLs carry most of the cholesterol in the blood, and if all of it is not removed from the blood, cholesterol and fat can build up in the arteries contributing to atherosclerosis. This is why LDL cholesterol is often called "bad" LDL cholesterol.

Q. Does an elevated total cholesterol or LDL cholesterol level increase my risk for having coronary heart disease?
A. Yes, if your total cholesterol level is:
- 200-239, you are classified as being "borderline high" and are at increased risk compared to those with lower levels.
- 240 and above, you have "high" cholesterol and your risk is even greater.

If your LDL cholesterol level is:
- 130 - 159, you are classified as being borderline high and are at increased risk compared to those with lower levels.
- 160 -189, you have a high LDL cholesterol and your risk increases.
- 190 and above, you have a very high level and medication may be needed along with diet to help lower it.

Q. What should my cholesterol levels be?
A. The desirable cholesterol levels are:
- Adults-- Total cholesterol less than 200
          LDL cholesterol 100 or less
          HDL cholesterol above 60
          Triglycerides less than 150

- Children--Total cholesterol less than 170
          LDL Cholesterol less than 110
          HDL cholesterol above 45
          Triglycerides less than 85

Q.What should I do to lower my high cholesterol levels?
A. Work with your doctor in doing the following things:
- Eat less high fat foods, especially ones high in saturated fat.
- Replace part of the saturated fat in your diet with mono-unsaturated fat
- Eat less high cholesterol foods.
- Choose foods high in complex carbohydrates, especially those high in soluble fiber.
- Do moderate exercise at least 20-30 mins. 4-5 times a week.
- Reduce your weight if over recommended weight.

Q. How long will it take to lower my cholesterol?

A. Generally your cholesterol level should begin to drop 2 to 3 weeks after you start on a cholesterol lowering program. How rapidly and how low it drops, depends on:

   a) How high it was to begin with
   b) How well you follow the program
   c) How responsive your body is to the cholesterol lowering program

Q. How long do I need to follow a program?

A. The program should be continued for life. While eating some foods high in saturated fat and cholesterol for one day or at one meal will not raise cholesterol levels, resuming old eating patterns, and putting on extra weight will.

Q. Will I need medication to lower my cholesterol?

A. Usually your doctor will have you follow a diet and exercise program for at least six months. If your cholesterol level has not dropped sufficiently, then you may be put on a medication along with your diet.

Q. Besides cutting down on saturated fat and cholesterol laden foods, which of the steps below can a person take to reduce the chances of suffering a heart attack or stroke?

   a) Regular physical activity/Exercise
   b) Stop smoking
   c) Keep blood pressure under control
   d) All of the above

A. High blood pressure and smoking increase the risk of having a heart attack. To reduce the overall risk, most doctors suggest:

   • If you don't exercise, start   • If you smoke, stop
   • If your blood pressure is high, endeavor to lower it.
Therefore "d" is the best answer.

Q. Are foods labeled "No Cholesterol" okay to buy and eat?

A. It depends. Many foods boasting "No Cholesterol" are high in saturated fat which is just as bad (if not worse for you) as cholesterol. Your best bet is to read the ingredient list on the label of the product to see what the fat content is.

Q. Is it ever too late to correct a cholesterol problem?
A. No! It is never too late to do something that may help your body chemistry function better and more efficiently.

Q. Is margarine safe to use if the label states, "Cholesterol Free"?
A. All margarines are "Cholesterol Free" because they are made from vegetable oils, not animal products. It's not a question of a food being safe or not, it's a matter of some foods being more beneficial than others in relation to the type of fat they contain, saturated or unsaturated. Use soft margarines which list an acceptable liquid vegetable oil first on the ingredient list. This indicates that the margarine is more unsaturated than saturated. If they say no trans fat that is even better. Also there are a couple of vegetable oil spreads (Take Control and Benacol) you can use which actually help lower an elevated LDL level. Only 2 to 3 tablespoons are to be used daily.

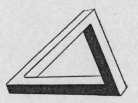

BIBLIOGRAPHY

Behram, Kliegman and Jenson. Nelson Textbook of Pediatrics, W. B. Saunders Co. 2000

Kavey, Rae-Ellen W., MD. "Hypercholesterolemia in Children." American Family Physician. Vol 61. no. 3, February, 1, 2000 633-635

Newman, Thomas B., MD, MPH and Garber, Alan M., MD. PhD. "Cholesterol Screening in Children and Adolescents." Pediatrics 2000; 105-638

"Practical Guide: Identification, Evaluation, and Treatment of Overweight and Obesity in Adults." U.S. Department of Health and Human Services, National Institutes of Health, National Heart, Lung and Blood Institute. NIH Pub. no. 00-4084, October, 2000

"Report of the Expert Panel on Blood cholesterol Levels in Children and Adolescents," U.S. Department of Health and Human Services, National Institutes of Health, National Heart, Lung and Blood Institute, National Cholesterol Education Program, September, 1991

Shamir, Raanan, MD and Fisher, Edward, MD. PhD. "Dietary Therapy for Children with Hypercholesterolemia." American Family Physician, vol. 61, no. 3 February 1, 2000, 675-682

Tanne, David, MD; Koren-Morag, Koren, PhD; Graff, Eran, PhD; Gold, Uri, PhD, for the BIP Study Group. "Blood Lipids and First-Ever Ischemic Stroke/Transient Ischemic Attack in the Bezafibrate Infarction Prevent (BIP) Registry." Circulation Journal , December 2001

"Third Report of the National Cholesterol Education Program Expert Panel on Detection, Evaluation, and Treatment of High Blood Cholesterol in Adults (Adult Treatment Pane III)." National Institutes of Health, National Heart, Lung and Blood Institute, May 2001

"Live Healthier, Live Longer; Lowering Cholesterol For the Person With Heart disease." National Institutes of Health, National Heart, Lung, and Blood Institute. NIH Pub. no. 96-3805, September, 1996

"Understanding and Controlling Cholesterol." American Heart Association, December, 1999

Valente, Anne Marie, MD; Newburger, Jane, MD, MPH and Lauer, Ronald, MD. "Hyperlipidemia in Children and adolescents." American Heart Journal, September 2001

COOKBOOK

When cooking to lower and control your cholesterol, remember it is most important to:

1. Avoid or decrease the saturated fat found mainly in:
   - meats
   - dairy foods
   - tropical oils
2. Decrease the total fat content of foods prepared
   - can use applesauce to replace part of vegetable oil in recipes
3. Prepare more complex carbohydrate foods:
   - whole grain cereals, pastas and breads
   - vegetables
   - fruits

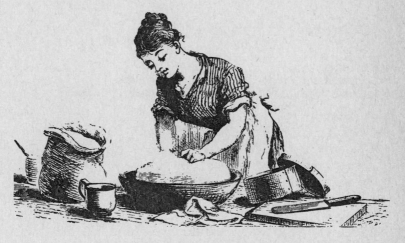

What did the dough say to the baker?
"It's nice to be kneaded."

BREAKFAST

Breakfast is the most important meal of the day. It is the source of energy for getting your day off to a good start. Children should get a quarter of their daily food energy needs at breakfast. Any wholesome food can be eaten for breakfast, it doesn't have to be "traditional" breakfast food. Even something left over from dinner the night before, such as chicken, fruit salad, or a whole grain muffin and nonfat/lowfat yogurt or a drink made from fresh fruit and nonfat/1% milk.

Forget syrup for topping whole grain pancakes and waffles. Excess sugar intake possibly increases the triglyceride level, a no, no. Try using fresh or frozen fruits pureed and applesauce.

If you enjoy cereal for breakfast, stay away from prepared granola because it is high in fat.

FRENCH TOAST
4 slices

Ingredients:
4 egg whites	1/2 tsp. vanilla
1/3 cup orange juice	4 slices whole wheat bread

Preparation:
In shallow dish, beat together:
  4 egg whites
  1/3 cup orange juice
  1/2 tsp. vanilla
Spray skillet with nonstick vegetable coating
Heat skillet to medium heat
Dip slices of bread in egg mixture to coat both sides
Place in skillet and brown both sides of bread
Serve with pureed fruit, fruit only preserves or
  unsweetened applesauce
Enjoy!

Estimated nutrition information per 2 slices:
Total fat	2.0 grams	Monounsaturated fat	0.8 grams
Saturated fat	0.8 grams	Polyunsaturated fat	0.6 grams
		Cholesterol	0 milligrams

APPLE, RAISIN OAT BRAN CEREAL
serves 2

Ingredients:

2 cups water	1/2 apple, diced
1/8 tsp. salt	2 Tbs. raisins
2/3 cup Quaker Oat Bran Cereal	1/2 tsp. cinnamon
	2 Tbs. wheat germ

Preparation:

Combine in saucepan:
2 cups water
1/8 tsp. salt
Oat bran cereal
diced apple
2 Tbs. raisins
1/2 tsp. cinnamon
Bring to boil over high heat

Reduce heat
Cook 1 minute, stirring occasionally

Divide between 2 serving bowls
Sprinkle with wheat germ
Serve with skim milk

Estimated nutrition information per serving:

Total fat	3.1 grams	Monounsaturated fat	1.4 grams
Saturated fat	0.2 grams	Polyunsaturated fat	1.4 grams
		Cholesterol	0 milligrams

OAT PANCAKES
serves 4

Ingredients:

4 egg whites	4 tsp. baking powder
2 Tbs. canola oil	1 tsp. cinnamon
1 3/4 cups orange juice	1/4 tsp. salt

2 cups oat flour (Grind rolled oats in blender to make oat flour)

Preparation:

Combine in medium bowl:
4 egg whites
2 Tbs. oil
1 3/4 cups orange juice

Combine in small bowl:
 2 cups flour
 4 tsp. baking powder
 1 tsp. cinnamon
 1/4 tsp. salt
Add to liquids, stir just until completely moistened
Cook on hot griddle on skillet, turning once
Delicious with applesauce

Estimated nutrition information per serving:

Total fat	9.8 grams	Monounsaturated fat	5.0 grams
Saturated fat	1.0 grams	Polyunsaturated fat	3.8 grams
		Cholesterol	0 milligram

CORNMEAL PANCAKES
serves 4

Ingredients:

1 1/2 cups cornmeal	2 egg whites
2 tsp. baking powder	2 Tbs. canola oil
1/4 tsp. salt	2 Tbs. concentrated fruit juice
	1 cup skim milk

Preparation:
Mix together in small bowl:
 1 1/2 cups cornmeal
 2 tsp. baking powder
 1/4 tsp. salt
Beat together in bowl until smooth:
 2 egg whites
 2 Tbs. canola oil
 2 Tbs. concentrated fruit juice
 1 cup skim milk

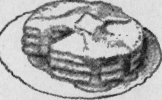

Add cornmeal mixture
Stir just till moistened
Cook on lightly oiled griddle until golden brown, turn once.
Serve with applesauce or fruit only preserves

Estimated nutrition information per serving:

Total fat	8.0 grams	Monounsaturated fat	4.1 grams
Saturated fat	0.6 grams	Polyunsaturated fat	2.7 grams
		Cholesterol	1 milligrams

WAFFLES
serves 3

Ingredients:
2 cups whole wheat pastry flour
3 tsp. baking powder
1 tsp. sugar
1/4 tsp. salt

1 3/4 cups skim milk
2 Tbs. canola oil
6 egg whites

Preparation:
Combine in medium bowl:
   2 cups flour
   3 tsp. baking powder
   1 tsp. sugar
   1/4 tsp. salt

Combine in small bowl:
   1 3/4 cups milk
   2 Tbs. canola oil
   4 egg whites
Add to above and mixed till smooth

Beat till stiff:
   2 egg whites
Fold into mixture

Pour 1/3 cup onto hot waffle grill and cook
Serve with pureed fruit, delicious

Estimated nutrition information per serving:

Total fat	6.8 grams	Monounsaturated fat	3.3 grams
Saturated fat	0.8 grams	Polyunsaturated fat	2.1 grams
		Cholesterol	3 milligrams

BANANA BREAKFAST DRINK
2 cups

Ingredients:
1 cup skim milk
1/3 cup nonfat dry milk
2 ripe bananas

1 tsp. vanilla
1 cup cracked ice
1/8 tsp. nutmeg

Preparation:
Place in blender:
1 cup skim milk
$1/3$ cup dry milk
2 ripe bananas, cut in chunks
1 tsp. vanilla
1 cup cracked ice
Blend until smooth
Pour into 2 glasses
Sprinkle with nutmeg

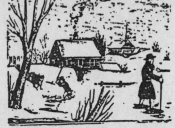

Serve with oat bran muffins

Estimated nutrition information per serving:

Total fat	1.6 grams	Monounsaturated fat	0.1 grams
Saturated fat	0.4 grams	Polyunsaturated fat	0.1 grams
		Cholesterol	5 milligrams

SCRAMBLED EGGS PLUS
serves 2

Ingredients:

1 egg + 4 egg whites	2 tsp. olive oil
1 Tbs. grated parmesan cheese	1 Tbs. chopped onion
2 Tbs. water	$1/4$ cup sliced mushrooms
salt & pepper	1 Tbs. chopped green pepper
$1/8$ tsp. basil	$1/2$ tomato, chopped

Preparation:
Combine in bowl:
eggs
1 Tbs. parmesan cheese
2 Tbs. water
salt & pepper to taste
$1/8$ tsp. basil, crushed

Saute in 2 tsp. olive oil in heavy skillet:
1 Tbs. chopped onion
$1/4$ cup sliced mushrooms
1 Tbs. chopped green pepper
$1/2$ tomato, chopped
Add egg mixture

Over medium heat, allow eggs to set slightly, pulling set edges inward and letting raw eggs flow out.
Continue scrambling to desired doneness.

Estimated nutrition information per serving:

Total fat	4.1 grams	Monounsaturated fat	1.3 grams
Saturated fat	1.4 grams	Polyunsaturated fat	0.4 grams
		Cholesterol	105 milligrams

OMELET GALORE
serves 3

Ingredients:

2 tsp. canola oil

$1/4$ cup chopped onions

3 Tbs. chopped green pepper

6 egg whites

$1/2$ tsp. marjoram

$1/4$ tsp. salt

dash pepper

$3/4$ cups diced cooked potatoes

2 Tbs. grated parmesan cheese

$3/4$ cup mung bean sprouts

Preparation:

Heat and saute in an oven broiler proof skillet:

2 tsp. canola oil

$1/4$ cup chopped onions

3 Tbs. green pepper

Combine in bowl:

6 egg whites

$1/2$ tsp. marjoram, crushed

$1/4$ tsp. salt

dash pepper

Pour over vegetables in skillet

Cook over low heat letting eggs set slightly then pulling the set edges inward to allow uncooked egg to flow to bottom.
When bottom of omelet is browned and top set:

arrange cooked potatoes on top

sprinkle with parmesan cheese

Place skillet under broiler

Cook until golden brown, about 1 minute

To serve, cut in 6 wedges, place bean sprouts on top each wedge

Estimated nutrition information per serving:

Total fat	4.4 grams	Monounsaturated fat	2.2 grams
Saturated fat	0.8 grams	Polyunsaturated fat	1.0 grams
		Cholesterol	3 milligrams

SOUPS

A bowl of hearty soup with an oat bran muffin and homemade chunky applesauce make a great meal on a cold winter evening.

To add variety to your soups, include vegetables that you would not ordinarily eat.

BEAN SOUP
8-10 cups

Ingredients:

1 lb. bag of mixed beans	1 1/2 tsp. dill weed
2 Tbs. broth or water	1/4 tsp. pepper
1 onion, chopped	6 whole cloves
1/2 green pepper, chopped	1 tsp. oregano
2 stalks celery with tops, chopped	10 oz. corn
2 tsp. paprika	1 lb. can of tomatoes
2 quarts of defatted stock or water	1 large potato, chopped
1 bay leaf	2 carrots, chopped

Preparation:

Place beans in large pot:
Cover with water to 2" above beans
Bring to boil, boil 2 minutes
Remove from heat, cover and let stand 1 hour

Saute in 2 Tbs. broth or water in dutch oven:
   1 chopped onion
   1/2 chopped green peppers
   2 stalks celery, chopped
   2 tsp. paprika
Add:
   2 quarts of stock or water
   drained beans
   1 bay leaf
   1 1/2 tsp. dill weed
   1/4 tsp. pepper
   6 cloves
   1 tsp. oregano

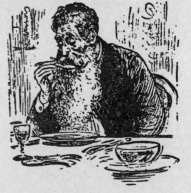

Simmer for 1-1 $1/2$ hours

Add:
10 oz. corn
1 lb. can tomatoes
1 chopped potato
2 chopped carrots

Simmer till vegetables and beans tender

If desire a thicker soup:
remove some potato and vegetables from soup
place in blender
blend till smooth
stir back into soup
For a fuller flavor, make a day ahead

Estimated nutrition information per serving, 1 cup

Total fat	2.4 grams	Monounsaturated fat	1.2 grams
Saturated fat	0.3 grams	Polyunsaturated fat	0.7 grams
		Cholesterol	0 milligrams

CORN CHOWDER DELIGHT
serves 8

Ingredients:

3 onions, diced	$1/2$ tsp. pepper
1 Tbs. olive oil	$1/4$ tsp. thyme
1 cup celery, chopped	32 oz. frozen corn
2 cups defatted broth or water	4 cups skim milk
6 potatoes, peeled and chopped	parsley (optional)
1 tsp. salt	paprika (optional)

Preparation:
Add to heated large saucepan or soup kettle and saute:
1 Tbs. olive oil
1 Tbs. water
3 diced onions
1 cup chopped celery

Add:
2 cups broth or water
6 chopped potatoes

1 tsp. salt
$1/2$ tsp. pepper
$1/4$ tsp. thyme
Cook until potatoes tender, about 15 minutes
Mash potatoes slightly
Add:
32 oz. corn
4 cups milk
Simmer but do not boil, until corn cooked, 5 to 10 minutes
Serve garnished with parsley and/or paprika

Estimated nutrition information per serving, 1 cup:

Total fat	2.6 grams	Monounsaturated fat	1.4 grams
Saturated fat	0.5 grams	Polyunsaturated fat	0.4 grams
		Cholesterol	3 milligrams

MINESTRONE
10-12 cups

Ingredients:

1 Tbs. olive oil
1 onion, chopped
1 1/2 cups celery, chopped
1 clove garlic, minced
1/2 cup chopped parsley
salt & pepper to taste
2 bay leaves
1 tsp. oregano
2 tsp. basil
1/2 tsp. rosemary
5 cups crushed tomatoes

1/4 cup barley
3 cups + of chopped vegetables;
 carrot, corn, green beans,
 green pepper, peas, potato
1 cup lima beans
1 cup canned garbanzo beans
1 cup whole wheat macaroni
1/4 cup chopped zucchini
1/4 cup chopped cabbage
1/4 cup sliced mushrooms
parmesan cheese

Preparation:

Heat in heavy soup pot:
3 Tbs. water
1 Tbs. olive oil

Add and saute until soft:
1 chopped onion
1 1/2 cups chopped celery
1 minced garlic clove

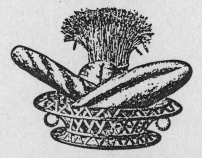

Add:
  $1/2$ cup chopped parsley
  salt & pepper to taste
  2 bay leaves
  1 tsp. oregano, crushed
  2 tsp. basil, crushed
  $1/2$ tsp. rosemary, crushed
  5 cups crushed tomatoes
  $1/4$ cup barley
Bring to boil over medium heat
Reduce heat and simmer while you prepare vegetables
Stir occasionally

Add:
  3 cups chopped vegetables
  1 cup lima beans
  1 cup garbanzo beans
  1 cup macaroni
  Bring to boil
Reduce heat and simmer until vegetables almost cooked
Stir occasionally
Add:
  $1/4$ cup chopped zucchini
  $1/4$ cup sliced mushrooms
  $1/4$ cup chopped cabbage
Simmer 5-10 minutes
Taste to check seasoning, adjusting as needed
If soup too thick, add some tomato juice, broth or water
Sprinkle each serving with 1 tsp. parmesan cheese

Estimated nutrition information per serving, 1 cup:

Total fat	3.5 grams	Monounsaturated fat	1.4 grams
Saturated fat	0.7 grams	Polyunsaturated fat	0.6 grams
		Cholesterol	1.5 milligrams

LENTIL SOUP
serves 4

Ingredients:

4 cups defatted stock or water
1 cup lentils
1/2 cup brown rice
salt to taste
1 tsp. basil
1/2 tsp. tarragon
1 Tbs. olive oil

1 onion, sliced
1 green pepper, diced
2 carrots, diced
2 stalks celery & leaves, diced
1 clove garlic, minced
1 lb. fresh or canned tomatoes
1 Tbs. miso (optional)

Preparation:

Put in 2 quart saucepan:
   4 cups stock or water
   1 cup lentils
   1/2 cup brown rice
   salt to taste
   1 tsp. basil, crushed
   1/2 tsp. tarragon, crushed
Simmer 45 minutes

Heat in soup pot:
   1 Tbs. oil
Saute:
   1 sliced onion
   1 diced pepper
   2 diced carrots
   2 stalks diced celery
   1 clove minced garlic
Add:
   1 can tomatoes
   rice and lentil mixture
Simmer 15 minutes
Add 5 minutes before serving: (opt.)
   1 Tbs. miso thoroughly mixed with 1/2 cup soup
Stir well, and do not let soup boil

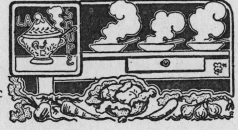

Estimated nutrition information per serving, 1 cup:
Total fat	4.9 grams	Monounsaturated fat	2.9 grams
Saturated fat	0.7 grams	Polyunsaturated fat	0.8 grams
		Cholesterol	0 milligrams

SALADS

SUNSHINE SALAD
serves 6

Ingredients:

1 3/4 cups orange juice
2 envelopes unflavored gelatin
2 Tbs. concentrated pineapple juice

1/4 cup lemon juice
1 1/2 cups carrots cut in 1"
   pieces
8 oz. crushed pineapple

Preparation:
   Pour into 5 cup blender:
      1/2 cup cold orange juice
   Sprinkle on top of juice and let stand 3-4 minutes:
      2 envelopes gelatin

   Heat and add to blender:
      1 1/4 cups orange juice
   Blend at low speed till gelatin completely dissolved, about 4
   minutes

   Add and blend at high speed till blended:
      2 Tbs. concentrated pineapple juice
      1/4 cup lemon juice

   Add and chop in blender:
      1 1/2 cups carrot pieces

   Pour into 8" square glass dish
   Stir in: 8 oz. crushed pineapple in own juice
   Chill till firm

Estimated nutrition information per serving:
   Total fat   0 grams   Monounsaturated fat 0 grams
   Saturated fat   0 grams   Polyunsaturated fat 0 grams
                                      Cholesterol   0 milligrams

WALDORF SALAD
serves 6

Ingredients:
3 medium apples, chopped
2 tsp. lemon juice
1/4 cup raisins
1/2 cup celery, chopped
1/4 cup chopped pecans
1/2 cup cut orange sections

1/4 cup plain low fat (1%) yogurt 1/8
2 tsp. brown sugar
1/8 tsp. cinnamon
1/8 sp. nutmeg
1 Tbs. sunflower seeds

Preparation:
Place in bowl:
    3 chopped apples
    2 tsp. lemon juice
Toss to coat apples
Add:
    1/4 cup raisins
    1/2 cup chopped celery
    1/4 cup chopped pecans
    1/2 cup cut oranges
Toss lightly to mix

Combine:
    1/4 cup plain yogurt
    2 tsp. brown sugar
    1/8 tsp. cinnamon
    1/8 tsp. nutmeg

Mix with fruit mixture
Toss together lightly
Chill
Serve on bed of lettuce
Sprinkle with sunflower seeds

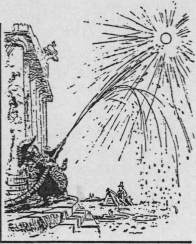

Estimated nutrition information per serving:

Total fat	3.9 grams	Monounsaturated fat	2.1 grams
Saturated fat	0.5 grams	Polyunsaturated fat	1.2 grams
		Cholesterol	1 milligram

CALICO SALAD
serves 6

Ingredients:

1 cup cooked potatoes, diced
1 cup cooked carrots, diced
1 cup cooked peas
1/4 cup red sweet pepper, chopped
1/4 cup cauliflower, chopped

2 Tbs. onions, chopped
2 Tbs. fresh parsley, chopped
1/4 cup light French dressing
1/2 head leaf lettuce

Preparation:
Combine in large bowl:
    all above ingredients except lettuce & dressing
Chill 1 hour

In another large bowl:
    break lettuce into bite-size pieces
Add:
    chilled vegetables
    dressing
Toss lightly

Estimated nutrition information per serving:

Total fat	1.5 grams	Monounsaturated fat	0.2 grams
Saturated fat	0.2 grams	Polyunsaturated fat	0.8 grams
		Cholesterol	0 milligrams

BEAN SALAD
serves 6

Ingredients:

1 carrot, sliced cooked crisp tender
16 oz can kidney or pink beans, drained
16 oz. can white beans, drained
1/4 cup green pepper, chopped
1/4 cup celery, sliced
2 Tbs. olive oil

2 Tbs. white wine vinegar
1/4 tsp. sugar
1/8 tsp. salt
1/8 tsp. oregano
1/8 tsp. basil
dash of pepper
Leaf lettuce for 6

Preparation:
Combine in bowl:
    1 cooked carrot
    2 cans beans
    1/4 cup choppedpepper
    1/4 cup sliced celery

Combine in small jar:
  2 Tbs. olive oil
  2 Tbs. white wine vinegar
  $1/4$ tsp. sugar
  $1/8$ tsp. salt
  $1/8$ tsp. oregano, crushed
  $1/8$ tsp. basil, crushed
  dash pepper
Cover and shake till thoroughly mixed
Pour over bean mixture
Toss to coat salad items

Cover, refrigerate at least 4 hours or overnight
Drain dressing from beans and reserve
Serve beans with lettuce
Serve reserved dressing to be used as desired

Estimated nutrition information per serving:

Total fat	4.9 grams	Monounsaturated fat	3.5 grams
Saturated fat	0.7 grams	Polyunsaturated fat	0.6 grams
		Cholesterol	0 milligrams

LENTIL SALAD
serves 4

Ingredients:

$1/2$ cup red lentils	1 Tbs. olive oil
1 Tbs. chopped scallions	1 $1/2$ tsp. tarragon vinegar
3 Tbs. fresh parsley, chopped	$1/4$ tsp. dry mustard
$1/4$ cup carrots, sliced thin	salt
green leaf lettuce	pepper
3 Tbs. broth or water	

Preparation:
Cook till tender, about 30 minutes:
  $1/2$ cup lentils in 1 $1/2$ cups water
Drain and cool lentils
Mix with cooled lentils:
  1 Tbs. chopped scallions
  3 Tbs. chopped parsley
  $1/4$ cup sliced carrots
Mix together in jar for dressing:
  3 Tbs. broth or water

1 Tbs. olive oil
1 1/2 tsp. tarragon vinegar
1/4 tsp. dry mustard
salt & pepper to taste
Shake well
Pour over lentil mixture
Chill
To serve, spoon onto bed of lettuce

Estimated nutrition information per serving:

Total fat	3.8 grams	Monounsaturated fat	2.6 grams
Saturated fat	0.5 grams	Polyunsaturated fat	0.4 grams
		Cholesterol	0 milligrams

VEGETABLE SALAD
serves 6-8

Ingredients:

1 1/2 lbs. broccoli
1 small head cauliflower
3 carrots, diagonally sliced, thin
1 can sliced beets, drained
1 red onion, sliced thin in rings
1 Tbs. olive oil

3 Tbs. tarragon vinegar
2 Tbs. broth or water
3 fresh basil leaves
2 garlic cloves, mashed
pepper
1 Tbs. dijon mustard

Preparation:

Separate broccoli flowerets from stems, cut stems on diagonal
   in 1/4" slices
Break cauliflower into pieces
Steam till crisp tender:
   1 1/2 lbs. broccoli
   1 head cauliflower
   3 carrots
Rinse under cold water
Put broccoli aside in refrigerator till later
Place in large bowl:
   carrots
   cauliflower
   1 can of beets
   1 onion cut in rings

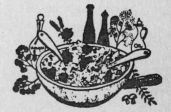

Combine in jar:
   1 Tbs. olive oil
   3 Tbs. tarragon vinegar

2 Tbs. broth or water
3 fresh basil leaves
2 mashed garlic cloves
pepper to taste
1 Tbs. mustard
Put on lid and shake well
Pour over vegetables in bowl, toss lightly

Cover and refrigerate 3-4 hours
Add broccoli $1/2$ hour before serving

Estimated nutrition information per serving:

Total fat	2.3 grams	Monounsaturated fat	1.3 grams
Saturated fat	0.3 grams	Polyunsaturated fat	0.4 grams
		Cholesterol	0 milligrams

CRANBERRY SALAD
serves 8

Ingredients:
1 envelope unflavored gelatin
1 $3/4$ cups apple juice
1 Tbs. sugar
2 cups fresh cranberries
1 tsp. orange rind
1 apple, chopped
$1/2$ cup celery, chopped
2 Tbs. lemon juice

Preparation:
Pour into saucepan:
$1/4$ cup apple juice
Sprinkle on juice:
1 envelope gelatin
Heat over medium heat, stirring till gelatin dissolves
Add 1 Tbs. sugar and stir till dissolved:
Add and mix well:
1 $1/2$ cups apple juice
2 cups chopped cranberries
1 tsp. orange rind
1 chopped apple
$1/2$ cup chopped celery
2 Tbs. lemon juice
Pour into mold
Chill till firm

Estimated nutrition information per serving:

Total fat	0 grams	Monounsaturated fat	0 grams
Saturated fat	0 grams	Polyunsaturated fat	0 grams
		Cholesterol	0 milligrams

ENTREES

The following entrees (main dishes) range from traditional meat and chicken dishes to not-so-familiar tofu (soybean product) dishes. You may wonder how you will be eating sufficient protein if there is no meat, poultry or fish as part of a meal. Grains, nuts & seeds (sesame, sunflower, etc) and legumes (beans, peas and lentils) all contain protein and when combined or served together make a complete protein. An excellent legume protein is tofu which comes from soybeans. It is high in protein, low in saturated fat and very versatile.

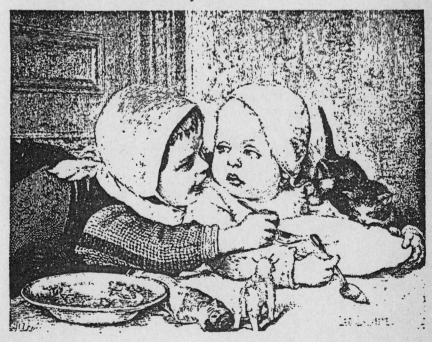

CHILI AND CORN
serves 6

Ingredients:

3 Tbs. vegetable broth or water	4 cups cooked kidney beans
1 onion, chopped	1/4 tsp. chili powder
1 clove garlic, minced	1/4 tsp. cumin powder
4 oz. can green chili peppers, diced	1 tsp. salt
2 cups crushed tomatoes	1 tsp. oregano
1 1/2 cups whole corn	1/2 tsp. dry mustard

Preparation:

Cook in Dutch oven till onion soft:

    3 Tbs. vegetable broth or water
    1 chopped onion
    1 minced garlic clove

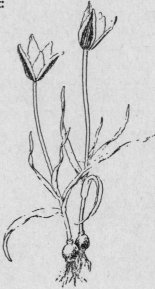

Add:

    4 oz. diced chili peppers
    2 cups crushed tomatoes
    1 1/2 cups corn
    4 cups cooked kidney beans
    1/4 tsp. chili powder
    1/4 tsp. cumin powder
    1 tsp. salt
    1 tsp. oregano, crushed
    1/2 tsp. dry mustard

Cover and simmer 30 minutes

If too thin:
remove some beans and blend in blender, stir back into chili
or
remove lid and cook about 10 minutes to reduce liquid

Estimated nutrition information per serving:

Total fat	0.7 grams	Monounsaturated fat	0.1 grams
Saturated fat	0.1 grams	Polyunsaturated fat	0.5 grams
		Cholesterol	0 milligrams

LASAGNA
serves 10-12

Ingredients:

5 1/4 cups Italian tomato sauce
6 Tbs. dried parsley
2 tsp. garlic powder
1 tsp. onion powder
1 1/4 tsp. oregano
1 1/4 tsp. basil

8 large whole wheat lasagna
   noodles
2 1/3 cups uncreamed low fat
   cottage cheese
1 cup nonfat buttermilk
3/4 cup grated sapsago cheese
4 egg whites, beaten stiffly

Preparation:

Combine in saucepan and cook 20-30 minutes:
   5 1/4 cups Italian tomato sauce
   2 Tbs. dried parsley
   2 tsp. garlic powder
   1 tsp. onion powder
   1 1/4 tsp. oregano
   1 1/4 tsp. basil
Begin heating water for cooking noodles
In bowl combine with fork:
   2 1/3 cups cottage cheese
   1 cup buttermilk
Add:
   3/4 cup grated sapsago cheese
   4 Tbs. parsley
Fold in:
   egg whites

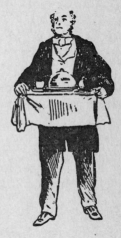

Refrigerate until noodles and sauce ready
Cook noodles according to package directions
Drain noodles
In a large shallow baking dish repeat layers of:
   tomato sauce
   noodles
   cheese mixture
   end with sauce on top
Bake at 375° about 1 hour, until thoroughly cooked and bubbly

Estimated nutrition information per serving, 1/12 of whole:

Total fat	2.6 grams	Monounsaturated fat	0.8 grams
Saturated fat	1.6 grams	Polyunsaturated fat	0.2 grams
		Cholesterol	13 milligrams

TOFU AND PEPPERS
serves 4

Ingredients:
2 Tbs. water or defatted broth
2 garlic cloves, minced
1/2 tsp. ground ginger
1 carrot cut in 1/4" slices
2 cups broccoli, cut in 1" pieces
1 sweet red pepper, cut in 1" pieces

1 green pepper, cut in 1" pieces
6 scallions, chopped
2 Tbs. soy sauce
1 Tbs. vinegar
1/2 lb. firm tofu, cut in small cubes

Preparation:
Heat in heavy skillet or wok:
   2 Tbs. water or defatted broth
Add:
   2 garlic cloves, minced
   1/2 tsp. ground ginger
   1 carrot cut in 1/4" slices
   2 cups broccoli, cut in 1" pieces
Stir-fry for 2-3 minutes

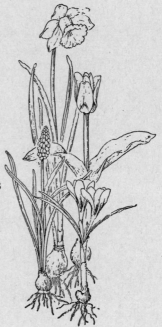

Add:
   1 sweet red pepper cut in 1" pieces
   1 green pepper cut in 1" pieces
Stir-fry for 3-4 minutes

Add:
   6 chopped scallions
Stir-fry 1 minute
Add and stir gently:
   2 Tbs. soy sauce
   1 Tbs. vinegar
   1/2 lb. cubed firm tofu
Cover and steam over low heat for 5-7 minutes

Enjoy with candle light and soft music

Estimated nutrition information per serving:

Total fat	3.7 grams	Monounsaturated fat	0.7 grams
Saturated fat	0.5 grams	Polyunsaturated fat	2.2 grams
		Cholesterol	0 milligrams

TOFU AND VEGETABLES, STIR-FRIED
serves 4-6

Ingredients:
2 Tbs. water or defatted broth
2 garlic cloves, minced
1/2 tsp. ginger
2 medium carrots, cut in thin slices
1 cup cut green beans
2 sweet red peppers, cut in 1" pieces

1 stalk celery, cut in 1" pieces
1 small onion, sliced
2 Tbs. soy sauce
2 tsp. vinegar
3/4 lb. tofu, cut in 1/2" cubes

Preparation:
Heat in large skillet or wok:
  2 Tbs. water or defatted broth

Add and stir fry for 2 minutes:
  2 garlic cloves, minced
  1/2 tsp. ginger
  2 medium carrots cut in thin slices
  1 cup cut green beans

Add and stir fry for 2 minutes:
  2 sweet red peppers, cut in 1" pieces
  1 stalk celery cut in 1" pieces

Add and stir fry 1 minute:
  1 small onion, sliced

Add and stir together:
  2 Tbs. soy sauce
  2 tsp. vinegar
  3/4 lb. tofu cut in 1 1/2" cubes
Cover and steam over low heat for 5-7 minutes

Serve immediately

Estimated nutrition information per serving, 1/6 of whole:

Total fat	3.3 grams	Monounsaturated fat	0.6 grams
Saturated fat	0.5 grams	Polyunsaturated fat	1.9 grams
		Cholesterol	0 milligrams

A fat kitchen, a lean will.--Benjamin Franklin, Poor Richard, 1733

SALMON AND ASPARAGUS WITH PASTA
serves 4

Ingredients:

1 tsp. canola oil
2 scallions, chopped
1 garlic clove, minced
1/2 tsp. fresh ginger, minced
1/2 can (14 oz.) water packed
   artichoke hearts, diced
1/2 cup defatted chicken broth
2 Tbs. fresh lemon juice

1 1/2 cups asparagus pieces or
   peas
6 1/2 oz. canned salmon, drained,
   rinsed, broken into large
   chunks
pepper to taste
1/2 lb. thin spinach spaghetti
4 tsp. Parmesan cheese

Preparation:

Begin heating water to cook pasta
Saute for 1 minute in 1 tsp. canola oil:
   2 chopped scallions
   1 minced garlic clove
   1/2 tsp. minced ginger
Add:
   1/2 can artichokes
   1/2 cup broth
   1 Tbs. lemon juice
Simmer 1 minute

Add and cook 2 to 4 minutes:
   1 1/2 cups cut asparagus or peas

Add and toss gently:
   canned salmon
Season with:
   pepper

Cook pasta according to directions
Drain and toss with:
   1 Tbs. lemon juice
Divide pasta among 4 plates
Top with salmon mixture
Sprinkle with Parmesan cheese

Estimated nutrition information per serving:

Total fat	5.7 grams	Monounsaturated fat	1.7 grams
Saturated fat	1.0 grams	Polyunsaturated fat	1.8 grams
		Cholesterol	19 milligrams

SHRIMP CREOLE
serves 4

Ingredients:

1 lb. cooked shrimp
2 Tbs. water
1/2 cup onions, chopped
1/2 cup green pepper, sliced thin
1/2 cup celery, diced
16 oz. tomato sauce
1 Tbs. vinegar
1 tsp. sugar

1/2 cup water
1/4 tsp. salt
pepper to taste
1 tsp. Worcestershire sauce
1/8 tsp. garlic powder
1/4 tsp. chili powder
1 bay leaf
1 Tbs. horseradish
2 cups cooked brown rice

Preparation:

Heat in large saucepan:
  2 Tbs. water
Add and saute till tender, stirring frequently:
  1/2 cup chopped onions
  1/2 cup sliced peppers
  1/2 cup diced celery
  add small amount of water if necessary to prevent drying
Add:
  16 oz. tomato sauce
  1 Tbs. vinegar
  1 tsp. sugar
  1/2 cup water
  1/4 tsp. salt
  pepper to taste
  1 tsp. Worcestershire sauce
  1/8 tsp. garlic powder
  1/4 tsp. chili powder
  1 bay leaf
  1 Tbs. horseradish

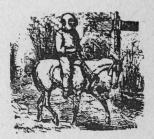

Heat until sauce just begins to boil, remove bay leaf
Reduce heat, add shrimp and heat through
Serve over brown rice

Estimated nutrition information per serving:

Total fat	2.0 grams	Monounsaturated fat	0.5 grams
Saturated fat	0.5 grams	Polyunsaturated fat	0.8 grams
		Cholesterol	171 milligrams

BAKED FLOUNDER
serves 2-4

Ingredients:

1 lb. fillets of flounder
1 tsp. canola oil
salt
pepper

paprika
$1/4$ tsp. thyme
2 Tbs. Swiss cheese (optional)

Preparation:

Place in lightly oiled baking dish:
   fillets
Brush with:
   1 tsp. canola oil

Sprinkle with:
   salt
   pepper
   paprika
   $1/4$ tsp. thyme
   2 Tbs. grated Swiss cheese (optional)
Bake at 400° for 10 to 15 minutes

Estimated nutrition information per serving:

Total fat	3.3 grams	Monounsaturated fat	1.1 grams
Saturated fat	1.0 grams	Polyunsaturated fat	0.9 grams
		Cholesterol	70 milligrams

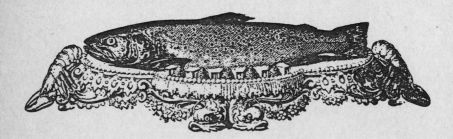

TURKEY CHILI
serves 10-12

Ingredients:

1 1/4 lb. ground turkey breast
2 large onions, chopped
2 15-19 oz. cans kidney beans
2 15-19 oz. cans pinto beans
1 28 oz. can peeled Italian tomatoes
1 14 1/2 oz. can stewed tomatoes

1 large green pepper, chopped
2-4 Tbs. chili powder
1 tsp. garlic powder
1 tsp. oregano
1/8 tsp. ground red pepper
1/8 tsp. pepper

Preparation:

Cook in Dutch Oven in 2 tsp. canola oil:
  ground turkey till brown
  2 chopped onions till tender
Drain off fat

Stir in:
  4 cans beans, reserve liquid to add later if desire thinner chili
  1 can cut up Italian tomatoes
  1 can stewed tomatoes
  1 chopped pepper
  2-4 Tbs. chili powder
  1 tsp. garlic powder
  1 tsp. oregano, crushed
  1/8 tsp. ground red pepper (optional)
  1/8 tsp. pepper

Bring to boil
Reduce heat, simmer uncovered for 1 1/4 hours or until desired
  consistency
Stir occasionally

Estimated nutrition information per serving:

Total fat	0.5 grams	Monounsaturated fat	0.1grams
Saturated fat	0.2 grams	Polyunsaturated fat	0.2grams
		Cholesterol	33 milligrams

TURKEY COLOMBO
serves 8

Ingredients:

1/3 cup oat or rice bran
1 tsp. oregano, crushed
1/4 tsp. garlic powder
1/4 tsp. onion powder
1/4 tsp. pepper, freshly ground
1 1/2 lbs. turkey cutlet, cut in
serving size pieces

1/2 cup skim milk
1/2 lb. fresh mushrooms, sliced
3 Tbs. tomato paste
1/4 cup marsala or sherry
2 Tbs. fresh parsley, chopped

Preparation:

Mix together in shallow dish:
1/3 cup oat or rice bran
1 tsp. crushed oregano
1/4 tsp. garlic powder
1/4 tsp. onion powder
1/4 tsp. pepper

Pour into another shallow dish:
1/2 cup skim milk
Dip turkey pieces into milk then into bran mixture
Broil until golden on both sides

Combine:
1/2 lb.sliced mushrooms
3 Tbs. tomato paste
1/4 cup wine
Pour over cutlets
Simmer 10 minutes
Serve garnished with parsley

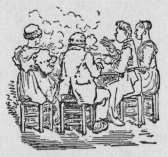

Estimated nutrition information per serving:

Total fat	3.3 grams	Monounsaturated fat	0.5 grams
Saturated fat	0.9 grams	Polyunsaturated fat	0.7 grams
		Cholesterol	59 milligrams

TURKEY STROGANOFF
serves 4

Ingredients:

1 lb. turkey breast slices
3/4 lb. fresh mushrooms, sliced
1 medium onion, sliced
1 green pepper, sliced thin
1 cup plain nonfat yogurt, room
  temp.

2 Tbs. flour
1/2 tsp. thyme
1/2 tsp. garlic salt
2 tsp. prepared mustard
1 tsp. prepared horseradish
paprika

Preparation:

Cut meat diagonally across grain in 1" wide strips
In skillet, brown strips quickly in:
  2 Tbs. water
Push browned meat to one side and add:
  3/4 lb.sliced mushrooms
  1 sliced onion
  1 sliced pepper
Cook till just tender
Combine:
  1 cup yogurt
  2 Tbs. flour
  1/2 tsp. thyme
  1/2 tsp. garlic salt
  2 tsp. prepared mustard
  1 tsp. prepared horseradish

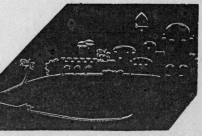

Add to skillet, stirring constantly till thickens slightly and
  bubbles
Serve over hot cooked noodles, sprinkle with paprika

Estimated nutrition information per serving:

Total fat	3.3 grams	Monounsaturated fat	0.5grams
Saturated fat	0.8 grams	Polyunsaturated fat	0.7 grams
		Cholesterol	59 milligrams

CHICKEN A LA KING
serves 4

Ingredients:

1 Tbs. canola oil

2 Tbs. chopped green pepper

2 Tbs. chopped onion

1/4 cup celery, diced

2 Tbs. flour

1/2 tsp. salt

2 cups skim or low fat milk

2 1/2 cups cooked chicken breast, chopped

2 Tbs. chopped pimentos

3/4 cup sliced mushrooms

Preparation:

Heat in skillet or stove top casserole:

 1 Tbs. canola oil

Add and saute lightly:

 2 Tbs. chopped green pepper

 2 Tbs. chopped onion

 1/4 cup diced celery

Stir in till well blended:

 2 Tbs. flour

 1/2 tsp. salt

Stir while adding:

 2 cups milk

Cook and stir until smooth and slightly thickened

Add:

 2 1/2 cups, chopped chicken

 2 Tbs. chopped red pimentos

 3/4 cup sliced mushrooms

Stir until well mixed

Heat thoroughly

May be served over:

 biscuits

 toast

 brown rice

 noodles

Eat and enjoy as if a king!

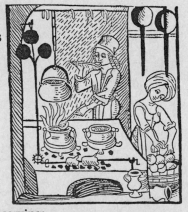

Estimated nutrition information per serving:

Total fat	7.1 grams	Monounsaturated fat	3.1 grams
Saturated fat	1.3 grams	Polyunsaturated fat	1.9 grams
		Cholesterol	76 milligrams

OVEN FRIED CHICKEN TERIYAKI
serves 12

Must be partly prepared the day before or morning of day served
Ingredients:

1 1/2 cups soya sauce (salt reduced)
2 1/2 cups unsweetened pineapple juice
2 1/4 tsp. garlic powder
1/2 cup cornmeal
1 tsp. onion powder
1/2 tsp. poultry seasoning

1 1/2 cups lemon juice
1 Tbs. ground ginger
6 large halved chicken breasts
1/2 cup oat bran
1/2 tsp. paprika
1/4 tsp. pepper
2 Tbs. sapsago cheese

Preparation:
Combine in shallow baking dish for marinade:
1 1/2 cups soya sauce
1 1/2 cups lemon juice
2 1/2 cups unsweetened pineapple juice
1 Tbs. ground ginger
1 1/2 tsp. garlic powder

Remove skin and fat from chicken, cut halved breast in half
Marinate chicken for several hours or over night in refrigerator

When ready to cook chicken, preheat oven to 350° & combine:
1/2 cup cornmeal
1/2 cup oat bran
1 tsp. onion powder
3/4 tsp. garlic powder
1/2 tsp. paprika
1/2 tsp. poultry seasoning
1/4 tsp. pepper
2 Tbs. grated sapsago cheese

Remove chicken from marinade
Coat well with cornmeal oat mixture
Arrange on nonstick baking sheet

Cover with aluminum foil, except for the first 10 and last 10 minutes of cooking, bake for 1 hour or until tender

Estimated nutrition information per serving:

Total fat	3.7 grams	Monounsaturated fat	1.1 grams
Saturated fat	0.9 grams	Polyunsaturated fat	0.7 grams
		Cholesterol	74 milligrams

VEGETABLES

Vegetables are complex carbohydrates and are excellent sources of soluble fiber. To retain their vitamins and minerals, try steaming vegetables rather than boiling them and throwing many of their nutrients down the drain with the cooking water.

DEVILED GREEN BEANS
serves 5

Ingredients:
1 lb. whole green beans
1/2 cup low fat plain yogurt
1 tsp. prepared mustard
Hot pepper sauce to taste

1 tsp. Worcestershire sauce
1/4 tsp. pepper
Cayenne pepper to taste

Preparation:
Cook beans and drain
Combine in small bowl:
   1/2 cup yogurt
   1 tsp. mustard
   hot pepper sauce to taste
   1 tsp. Worcestershire sauce
   1/4 tsp. pepper
   Cayenne pepper to taste
Pour over hot beans, serve immediately
Hm-Hm Good!

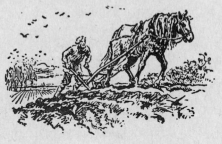

Estimated nutrition information per serving:

Total fat	0.7 grams	Monounsaturated fat	0.1 grams
Saturated fat	0.3 grams	Polyunsaturated fat	0.2 grams
		Cholesterol	1 milligram

PICKLED BEETS
serves 4

Ingredients:
1 lb. beets
1/4 cup vinegar
1/8 tsp. salt
4 cloves

1/4 tsp. mustard seeds
1 tsp. prepared mustard
1/2 tsp. basil, crushed
dash of pepper

Preparation:
Slip into boiling water:
  scrubbed beets
Cook till tender, about 30 to 40 minutes
Hold cooked beet under running cool water and slip off its skin
While beets cooking, combine:
  1 cup water
  1/4 cup vinegar
  1/8 tsp. salt
  4 cloves
  1/4 tsp. mustard seeds
  1 tsp. prepared mustard
  1/2 tsp. crushed basil
  dash of pepper
Slice cooked beets into shallow dish
Pour vinegar mixture over beets
Chill for at least 3 hours

Estimated nutrition information per serving:

Total fat	0 grams	Monounsaturated fat	0 grams
Saturated fat	0 grams	Polyunsaturated fat	0 grams
		Cholesterol	0 milligrams

GREEN BEANS AND TOMATOES
serves 6

Ingredients:

20 oz. whole green beans
1 Tbs. water or broth
$1/2$ cup onion, chopped
4 medium tomatoes, chopped

$1/8$ tsp. salt
$1/2$ tsp. marjoram, crushed
1 tsp. tarragon, crushed

Preparation:

Cook in saucepan:
   20 oz. beans

Add to skillet over medium heat:
   1 Tbs. water or broth
   $1/2$ cup chopped onions
Cook 5 minutes
Add:
   4 chopped tomatoes
   $1/8$ tsp. salt
   $1/2$ tsp. crushed marjoram
   1 tsp. crushed tarragon
Cover and simmer 10 minutes

Add:
   cooked beans
Cover, simmer till thoroughly heated

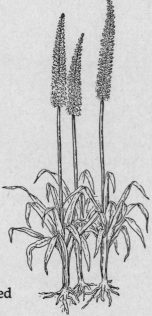

Estimated nutrition information per serving:

Total fat	0 grams	Monounsaturated fat	0 grams
Saturated fat	0 grams	Polyunsaturated fat	0 grams
		Cholesterol	0 milligrams

BAKED SQUASH
serves 3-4

Ingredients:

1 acorn squash
1 tsp Olive oil
1 $1/4$ cups applesauce

2 tsp. brown sugar
Cinnamon

Preparation:
  Wash, cut in half, remove seeds from:
  1 squash
  Rub cut area with olive oil
  Place cut side down in glass baking dish:
  Bake at 350° for 35 minutes

  Turn squash over and continue baking for 25 minutes or till
    tender
  Heat in saucepan:
    applesauce
  Sprinkle on inside of squash when it is baked:
    2 tsp. brown sugar
    cinnamon to taste
  Spoon into squash:
    hot applesauce

Variation: May remove cooked squash from shell and mix all
ingredients together, then serve.

Estimated nutrition information per serving:

Total fat	1.17 grams	Monounsaturated fat	0.85 grams
Saturated fat	0.15 grams	Polyunsaturated fat	0.4 grams
		Cholesterol	0.1 milligrams

CARROTS, CAULIFLOWER AND PEPPERS
serves 4

Ingredients:
  2 Tbs. broth or water
  2 cups carrots, diagonally cut
  1/4 cup green bell pepper, chopped

  2 cups cauliflower, small pieces
  1/4 tsp. tarragon, crushed
  1/4 tsp. rosemary, crushed

Preparation:
  Heat in heavy skillet over med-high heat:
    2 Tbs. broth or water
  Add, stir for 2 minutes:
    2 cups cut carrots
  Add, stir 1 minute:
    1/4 cup chopped peppers

Add, stir 2 minutes:
  2 cups cut cauliflower
  1/4 tsp. crushed tarragon
  1/4 tsp. crushed rosemary
Cover and cook over low heat about 10 minutes or till
  vegetables tender

Estimated nutrition information per serving:
Total fat	0.2 grams	Monounsaturated fat	0.0 grams
Saturated fat	0.1 grams	Polyunsaturated fat	0.1 grams
		Cholesterol	0 milligrams

CHEESY CAULIFLOWER
serves 4

Ingredients:

3 cups cauliflower flowerets
1/2 cup low fat cottage cheese
1 tsp. lemon juice
1 tsp. red wine vinegar
1 tsp. onion, minced

2 Tbs. fresh parsley, chopped
1 Tbs. Parmesan cheese, grated
1/4 tsp. dry mustard
1/4 tsp. dill weed
1 tsp. paprika

Preparation:
Steam till tender, about 10 minutes:
  cauliflower flowerets
Combine, blend in blender till smooth:
  1/2 cup cottage cheese
  1 tsp. lemon juice
  1 tsp. red wine vinegar
  1 tsp. minced onion
  2 Tbs. chopped parsley
  1 Tbs. grated Parmesan cheese
  1/4 tsp. dry mustard
  1/4 tsp. dill weed
Pour over cauliflower
Sprinkle with:
  1 tsp. paprika

Estimated nutrition information per serving:
Total fat	0.8 grams	Monounsaturated fat	0.2 grams
Saturated fat	0.4 grams	Polyunsaturated fat	0.1 grams
		Cholesterol	3 milligrams

TASTY CABBAGE
serves 4

Ingredients:

1 Tbs. water

3 cups cabbage, shredded

1 cup celery, chopped

1 cup red bell pepper, chopped

$3/4$ cup onion, chopped

$1/4$ tsp. salt

$1/4$ tsp. savory

dash pepper

Preparation:

Heat in large skillet over medium heat:

1 Tbs. water

Combine and place in skillet:

3 cups chopped cabbage

1 cup chopped celery

1 cup chopped red bell pepper

$3/4$ cup chopped onion

$1/4$ tsp. salt

$1/4$ tsp. savory

dash pepper

Stir well

Cover, cook 5 minutes stirring occasionally

Serve immediately

Estimated nutrition information per serving:

Total fat	0 grams	Monounsaturated fat	0 grams
Saturated fat	0 grams	Polyunsaturated fat	0 grams
		Cholesterol	0 milligrams

SWEET & SOUR BROCCOLI
serves 5

Ingredients:

1 lb. broccoli flowerets

2 tsp. soft margarine

1 Tbs. brown sugar

3 Tbs. vinegar

$1/8$ tsp. dry mustard

$1/4$ cup onion, chopped

Preparation:

Cook broccoli, drain

Combine in small saucepan:

2 tsp. soft margarine

1 Tbs. brown sugar

3 Tbs. vinegar
$1/8$ tsp. dry mustard
$1/4$ chopped onion
Heat till hot

Pour over cooked, drained broccoli
Serve immediately

Estimated nutrition information per serving:

Total fat	1.6 grams	·	Monounsaturated fat	0.5 grams
Saturated fat	0.3 grams		Polyunsaturated fat	0.7 grams
			Cholesterol	0 milligrams

PEAS, MUSHROOMS AND TOMATOES
serves 6

Ingredients:

1 medium onion, sliced	$1/2$ lb. fresh whole mushrooms
$3/4$ tsp. ground turmeric	2 tsp. fresh lemon juice
$1/4$ tsp. ground ginger	$1/4$ tsp. salt
1 10 oz. package frozen peas,	2 medium tomatoes, cut in wedges

Preparation:
Cook and stir in skillet over medium heat till onion tender:
1 sliced onion
$3/4$ tsp. turmeric
$1/4$ tsp. ginger
2 Tbs. water

Stir in:
10 oz. peas
$1/2$ lb. whole mushrooms
2 tsp. lemon juice
$1/4$ tsp. salt
Cook uncovered, stirring occasionally till peas tender, about 3-5
minutes
Stir in tomato wedges
Heat just till hot

Estimated nutrition information per serving:

Total fat	0.2 grams	Monounsaturated fat	0.0 grams
Saturated fat	0.0 grams	Polyunsaturated fat	0.1 grams
		Cholesterol	0 milligrams

VEGETABLE STUFFED PEPPERS
serves 6

Ingredients:

6 medium green peppers
1 1/2 cups corn
1 cup diced tomatoes
1/2 cup soft, whole grain bread crumbs
1/3 cup celery, finely chopped

1 Tbs. light vegetable oil spread
2 Tbs. minced onion
3 egg whites, slightly beaten
1/4 tsp. salt
1/4 tsp. basil, crushed
dash pepper

Preparation:

Remove tops and seeds from peppers
Combine in bowl:
  1 1/2 cups corn
  1 cup diced tomatoes
  1/2 cup bread crumbs
  1/3 cup chopped celery
  1 Tbs. light vegetable oil spread
  2 Tbs. minced onions
  3 slightly beaten egg whites
  1/4 tsp. salt
  1/4 tsp. basil
  dash pepper
Stuff peppers with mixture

Place peppers upright in greased baking dish
Add:
  small amount of water
Cover, bake at 350° for 1 hour

Estimated nutrition information per serving:

Total fat	0.8 grams	Monounsaturated fat	0.4 grams
Saturated fat	0.08 grams	Polyunsaturated fat	0.3 grams
		Cholesterol	0 milligrams

STUFFED POTATOES
serves 4

Ingredients:
2 large baking potatoes, scrubbed
3/4 cup buttermilk
1/2 clove garlic
2 tsp. onion, minced

1/4 tsp. pepper
1/4 cup chives
1/4 cup skim milk mozzarella
   cheese, shredded
paprika

Preparation:
Bake potatoes till tender
Remove potatoes from oven
Cut in half lengthwise
Scoop out pulp

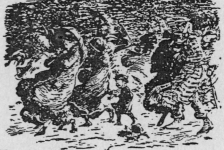

Place in blender:
  potato pulp
  3/4 cup buttermilk
  1/2 clove garlic
  2 tsp. minced onion
  1/4 tsp. pepper
  1/4 cup chives
  1/4 cup shredded cheese
Blend till fluffy and light

Spoon mixture back into potato shells
Sprinkle with paprika

Place potatoes under broiler till tops golden brown

Estimated nutrition information per serving:

Total fat	1.7 grams	Monounsaturated fat	0.5 grams
Saturated fat	1.1 grams	Polyunsaturated fat	0.1 grams
		Cholesterol	5 milligrams

"HOT" ZUCCHINI
serves 4-6

Ingredients:

2 Tbs. water or broth
1 lb. (4 cups) zucchini, sliced thin
1 cup carrots, shredded
1 large onion, chopped
$3/4$ cup celery, chopped
$1/2$ medium green pepper,
cut in thin strips
$1/4$ tsp. salt
$1/4$ tsp. garlic powder

$1/2$ tsp. dried basil, crushed
$1/2$ tsp. pepper
$1/3$ cup tomato sauce
$1/4$ tsp. chili powder
1 tsp. vinegar
1 tsp. hot sauce
1 Tbs. prepared mustard
2 tomatoes, cut in wedges

Preparation:

Heat in large skillet:
2 Tbs. water or broth
Add and mix together well:
4 cups sliced zucchini
1 cup shredded carrots
1 chopped onion
$3/4$ cup chopped celery
$1/2$ pepper cut in strips
$1/4$ tsp. salt
$1/4$ tsp. garlic powder
$1/2$ tsp. crushed basil
$1/8$ tsp. pepper
Cover, cook over med-high heat for 5 minutes, stir
occasionally
Combine and stir into vegetables:
$1/3$ cup tomato sauce
$1/4$ tsp. chili powder
1 tsp. vinegar
1 tsp. hot sauce
1 Tbs. prepared mustard
Add: tomato wedges
Cook uncovered 3-5 minutes or till thoroughly heated

Estimated nutrition information per serving:

Total fat	0.4 grams	Monounsaturated fat	0.0 grams
Saturated fat 0.1 grams		Polyunsaturated fat	0.2 grams
		Cholesterol	0 milligrams

VEGETABLE CASSEROLE
serves 6-8

Ingredients:

1 medium cauliflower head	1 tsp. curry powder
1 eggplant	$1/4$ tsp. salt
2 potatoes	$1/4$ tsp. turmeric powder
1 Tbs. canola oil	1 cup peas
1 tsp. mustard seed	1 tomato, finely chopped
	juice of 1 lemon

Preparation:

Remove:
   stem of cauliflower, cut into small pieces
Separate:
   flowerets, slice
Cut into $1/2$" cubes:
   eggplant
Cube and boil till partially cooked:
   2 potatoes
Heat in Dutch oven:
   1 Tbs. canola oil
Add and brown, covered:
   1 tsp. mustard seed
Stir in:
   1 tsp. curry powder
   $1/4$ tsp. salt
   $1/4$ tsp. turmeric powder
Add and stir to coat with spices and oil:
   cut cauliflower
Add:
   $1/4$ cup water
   cubed eggplant
   partially cooked potatoes
Continue cooking till almost desired doneness
Add 1 to 2 Tbs. water as needed, stirring gently
Add 5 minutes before serving:
   1 cup peas
When vegetables are cooked, stir in:
   chopped tomato
Turn off heat
Add lemon juice   Serve and enjoy

Estimated nutrition information per serving:

Total fat	1.9 grams	Monounsaturated fat	1.0 grams
Saturated fat	0.1 grams	Polyunsaturated fat	0.7 grams
		Cholesterol	0 milligrams

DRESSINGS AND DIPS

MOCK SOUR CREAM
1 cup

Ingredients:
- 1 cup nonfat plain yogurt
- 1 Tbs. chives, fresh or frozen

Preparation:
Mix yogurt and chives together
Serve with baked potatoes

Estimated nutrition information per serving, 1 Tbs.:

Total fat	0 grams	Monounsaturated fat	0.8 grams
Saturated fat	0 grams	Polyunsaturated fat	0.1 grams
		Cholesterol	1 milligram

or

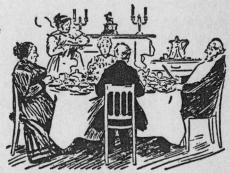

Ingredients:
- 1 cup low fat cottage cheese
- 2 Tbs. skim buttermilk
- 1 tsp. lemon juice

Preparation:
Place into blender:
- cottage cheese
- buttermilk
- lemon juice

Blend till smooth

Estimated nutrition information per serving, 1 Tbs.:

Total fat	0.1 grams	Monounsaturated fat	0.0 grams
Saturated fat	0.1 grams	Polyunsaturated fat	0.1 grams
		Cholesterol	1 milligram

MAYONNAISE
1 cup

Ingredients:

2/3 cup skim milk

2 Tbs. flour

1 large egg, room temperature

1/2 tsp. dry mustard

1/4 tsp. paprika

1/4 tsp. salt

1/8 tsp. cayenne pepper

2 Tbs. fresh lemon juice

1 Tbs. olive oil

Preparation:

Put in jar and shake till mixed:

1/3 cup cold milk

2 Tbs. flour

Pour into top of double boiler over low heat and add:

1/3 cup milk

Mix together

Stir in:

1 egg

1/2 tsp. dry mustard

1/4 tsp. paprika

1/4 tsp. salt

1/8 tsp. cayenne pepper

Cook over just simmering water, stirring constantly till thickened and smooth

Remove from heat and stir in:

2 Tbs. lemon juice

1 Tbs. olive oil

Cool and refrigerate in tightly covered container

Estimated nutrition information per serving, 1 Tbs.:

Total fat	1.3 grams	Monounsaturated fat	0.8 grams
Saturated fat	0.2 grams	Polyunsaturated fat	0.1 grams
		Cholesterol	17 milligrams

DILL AND YOGURT DRESSING
1 cup

Ingredients:
1 cup plain low fat yogurt

$1/2$ tsp. dill weed, crushed

2 tsp. onion, minced

1 tsp. lemon juice

2 tsp. finely chopped fresh parsley

$1/4$ tsp. dry mustard

$1/8$ tsp. garlic powder

Preparation:
Combine in small bowl:
  All above ingredients
Cover, refrigerate for several hours to blend flavors

Estimated nutrition information per serving, 2 Tbs.:

Total fat	0.5 grams	Monounsaturated fat	0.1 grams
Saturated fat	0.3 grams	Polyunsaturated fat	0 grams
		Cholesterol	2 milligrams

RUSSIAN SOUR CREAM DRESSING
about 2 cups

Ingredients:
3 hard boiled egg whites, chopped

1 cup low fat (1%) yogurt

2 Tbs. lemon juice

1 Tbs. drained capers

2 gherkin pickles, minced

salt

pepper

Preparation:
Mix all above ingredients together
Refrigerate at least 1 hour before using

Estimated nutrition information per serving, 1 Tbs.:

Total fat	0.1 grams	Monounsaturated fat	0 grams
Saturated fat	0.1 grams	Polyunsaturated fat	0 grams
		Cholesterol	0 milligrams

CHILI BEAN DIP
about 1 1/3 cup

Ingredients:

15 oz. can kidney beans
3 Tbs. bean liquid
1 Tbs. vinegar
1 tsp. chili powder

1/8 tsp. ground cumin
2 tsp. onion, grated
2 tsp. parsley, chopped

Preparation:

Drain:
    1 can kidney beans, reserve liquid
Place in blender:
    beans
    3 Tbs. bean liquid
    1 Tbs. vinegar
    1 tsp. chili powder
    1/8 tsp. ground cumin
Blend till smooth
Remove from blender and stir in:
    2 tsp. grated onion
    2 tsp. chopped parsley
Chill thoroughly
Serve with raw vegetable sticks

Estimated nutrition information per serving, 1 Tbs.:

Total fat	0.2 grams	Monounsaturated fat	0 grams
Saturated fat	0 grams	Polyunsaturated fat	0.1 grams
		Cholesterol	0 milligrams

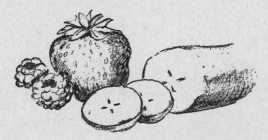

DESSERTS

Dessert is the end of the meal pleasure that should be eaten in a small quantity and savored. For low fat content, fruits, gelatins, puddings, and sherbet are at the top of the list. Be careful of cookies, cakes, cobblers and pies with pies having the highest fat content because of the fat in the crust.

GOOD OLD RICE PUDDING
serves 6

Ingredients:

4 cups 1% milk
1/4 cup brown rice
2 Tbs. sugar
1/4 tsp. salt
1/4 cup raisins
1/4 tsp. nutmeg

Preparation:

Combine in bowl:
4 cups milk
1/4 cup rice
2 Tbs. sugar
1/4 tsp. salt
Pour into lightly oiled 1 1/2 quart baking dish
Bake at 300° for 1 hour, stir frequently (every 15-20 minutes)
Stir in:
1/4 cup raisins
Sprinkle on top:
1/4 tsp. nutmeg
Continue baking 1 1/2 hours
Remove from oven, place on rack to cool

May be served warm or cold
When first removed from oven, may seem runny, but by time it has cooled, milk will have either thickened or become absorbed.

Estimated nutrition information per serving:

Total fat	1.5 grams	Monounsaturated fat	0.5 grams
Saturated fat	1.0 grams	Polyunsaturated fat	0.1 grams
		Cholesterol	7 milligrams

APPLE COOKIES
about 5 dozen small

Ingredients:
1 cup whole wheat pastry flour
$3/4$ cup oat bran
$1/2$ tsp. salt
$3/4$ tsp. baking powder
$1/2$ tsp. baking soda
$3/4$ tsp. cinnamon
$1/2$ tsp. ground cloves
$1/2$ tsp. cardamon (optional)

$1/2$ cup walnuts, chopped
$1/4$ cup concentrated pineapple juice
$1/3$ cup light olive oil
4 egg whites
1 cup rolled oats
2 large apples, chopped
$1/2$ cup raisins
$1/2$ cup dried apricots, chopped

Preparation:
Stir together in small bowl:
   1 cup whole wheat flour
   $3/4$ cup oat bran
   $1/2$ tsp. salt
   $3/4$ tsp. baking powder
   $1/2$ tsp. baking soda
   $3/4$ tsp. cinnamon
   $1/2$ tsp. cloves
   $1/2$ tsp. cardamon (optional)
   $1/2$ cup chopped walnuts
Beat together in large bowl:
   $1/2$ cup concentrated pineapple juice
   $1/3$ cup light olive oil
Beat in:
   4 egg whites
Stir in:
   flour mixture
   1 cup rolled oats
   2 chopped apples
   $1/2$ cup raisins
   $1/2$ cup chopped apricots
Mix well
Drop by teaspoon, 2" apart onto lightly greased cookie sheet
Bake at 350° 12-15 minutes

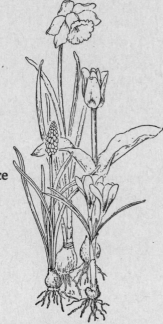

Estimated nutrition information per cookie:

Total fat	2.0 grams	Monounsaturated fat	1.1 grams
Saturated fat	0.2 grams	Polyunsaturated fat	0.6 grams
		Cholesterol	0 milligrams

RAISIN OATMEAL COOKIES
4 dozen

Ingredients:

1 1/2 cups whole wheat pastry flour
1/2 cup oat bran
1 tsp. baking soda
1/2 tsp. salt
1 tsp. cinnamon
1/4 + 1/8 tsp. cloves
1/4 + 1/8 tsp. nutmeg
3 cups rolled oats

4 egg whites, slightly beaten
1/4 cup concentrated pineapple
   juice
1/2 cup apples, chopped
1/2 cup canola oil
1/2 cup skim milk
1/2 cup orange juice
2 tsp. vanilla
2 cup raisins

Preparation:

Stir together with fork in bowl:
   1 1/2 cups flour
   1/2 cup oat bran
   1 tsp. baking soda
   1/2 tsp. salt
   1 tsp. cinnamon
   1/4 + 1/8 tsp. cloves
   1/4 + 1/8 tsp. nutmeg
   3 cups rolled oats
Combine in small bowl:
   4 beaten egg whites
   1/4 cup concentrated pineapple juice
   1/2 cup chopped apples
   1/2 cup canola oil
   1/2 cup skim milk
   1/2 cup orange juice
   2 tsp. vanilla
   2 cups raisins
Add to flour mixture
Mix well

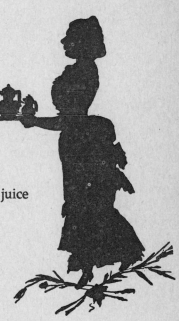

Place teaspoons of batter on lightly oiled cookie sheet
Bake at 375° 12-15 minutes
Bake shorter time for chewy cookie and longer for crisp cookie

Estimated nutrition information per cookie:

Total fat	2.5 grams	Monounsaturated fat	1.3 grams
Saturated fat	0.2 grams	Polyunsaturated fat	0.8 grams
		Cholesterol	0 milligrams

CHOCOLATE COOKIES
3 dozen cookies

Ingredients:
$1/3$ cup + 1 Tbs. canola oil

$1/3$ cup + 2 Tbs. sugar

2 egg whites, beaten

6 Tbs. cocoa

$1 3/4$ cups minus 1 Tbs. whole wheat pastry flour

$2 1/4$ tsp. baking powder

$1/4$ tsp. salt

$1/2$ cup skim milk

$1 1/2$ tsp. vanilla

Preparation:
Cream together in small bowl:

$1/3$ cup + 1 Tbs. canola oil

$1/3$ cup + 2 Tbs. sugar

Beat in:

2 egg whites

Combine:

6 Tbs. cocoa

$1 3/4$ cups flour minus 1 Tbs.

$2 1/4$ tsp. baking powder

$1/4$ tsp. salt

Add egg mixture to dry mixture alternately with:

$1/2$ cup milk

Mix well, stir in:

$1 1/2$ tsp. vanilla

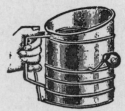

Using teaspoon, drop batter 2" apart onto lightly oiled cookie sheet

Bake at 400° for 8 to 10 minutes

Estimated nutrition information per cookie:

Total fat	2.5 grams	Monounsaturated fat	1.3 grams
Saturated fat	0.2 grams	Polyunsaturated fat	0.9 grams
		Cholesterol	0 milligrams

ANGEL FOOD CAKE
serves 12

Ingredients:
1 cup sifted whole wheat
  pastry flour
$1/2$ cup superfine sugar
$1 1/2$ cups (12) egg whites

1 1/2 tsp. cream of tartar
$1/4$ tsp. salt
2 tsp. vanilla

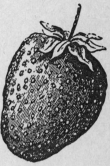

Preparation:
Sift together 4 times:
  1 cup flour
  $1/4$ cup sugar

Beat till stiff enough to hold soft peaks:
  $1 1/2$ cups egg whites
  $1 1/2$ tsp. cream of tartar
  $1/4$ tsp. salt
  2 tsp. vanilla
Add 1 Tbs. at a time, beat after each addition:
  $1/4$ cup sugar
Sift over egg whites:
  $1/4$ cup flour mixture at a time, fold in after each   addition
Place batter into 10" clean, ungreased tube pan
Gently cut with knife through batter in ever-widening circles to
  break air bubbles
Bake at 375° for 35-40 minutes
Remove from oven, invert pan till cake cool
Remove from pan

Estimated nutrition information per serving:

Total fat	trace grams	Monounsaturated fat	0 grams
Saturated fat	0 grams	Polyunsaturated fat	0 grams
		Cholesterol	0 milligrams

SOFT STRAWBERRY ICE CREAM
serves 4

Ingredients:
2 cups 1% milk
2 cups frozen strawberries
$1 1/2$ tsp. vanilla

2 Tbs. concentrated pineapple juice
$1/2$ cup dry low fat milk powder

Preparation:
  Blend above ingredients in blender till thick and smooth
  Serve immediately for soft ice cream
  or
  Freeze in ice cube trays, stirring once before freezing
    completed

Estimated nutrition information per serving:

Total fat	1.1 grams	Monounsaturated fat	0.4 grams
Saturated fat	0.8 grams	Polyunsaturated fat	0.2 grams
		Cholesterol	7 milligrams

FRUIT SHERBET
serves 4

Ingredients:
  1 cup plain nonfat yogurt
  1 Tbs. concentrated orange juice
  1/2 cup orange juice
  2 cups fresh or frozen strawberries

  1 lb. can crushed pineapple in
    own juice
  1/2 cup low fat milk powder
  1 banana, cut in chunks
  1 Tbs. lemon juice

Preparation:
  Blend together till smooth:
    all above ingredients
  Freeze in ice cube trays or other container
  Beat once before freezing completed

Estimated nutrition information per serving:

Total fat	0.4 grams	Monounsaturated fat	0.0 grams
Saturated fat	0.2 grams	Polyunsaturated fat	0.0 grams
		Cholesterol	3 milligrams

WHIPPED CREAM
3 cups

Ingredients:
  12 oz can evaporated skimmed milk
  2 Tbs. + 1 1/2 tsp. lemon juice

  1 Tbs. vanilla
  1 Tbs. sugar

Preparation:
Chill milk thoroughly in can
Shake can well, then pour milk into cold bowl
Whip with cold beaters
When milk very stiff, beat in:
2 Tbs. + 1 1/2 tsp. lemon juice (insures stiffness)
1 Tbs. vanilla
1 Tbs. sugar
Refrigerate till ready to use

Estimated nutrition information per 1/4 cup:

Total fat	0.1 grams	Monounsaturated fat	0.0 grams
Saturated fat	0.1 grams	Polyunsaturated fat	0.0 grams
		Cholesterol	1 milligrams

APPLE RASPBERRY WITH PEACHES
serves 6-8

Ingredients:
2 envelopes plain gelatin
1/2 cup cold water
3 cups Apple Raspberry juice
2 large fresh peaches, sliced
1 cup fresh Bing cherries, pitted
and cut in half

Preparation:
Sprinkle:
2 envelopes gelatin
On:
1/2 cup cold water in small saucepan
Heat, stirring constantly, until gelatin dissolves completely
Add to:
3 cups Apple Raspberry juice
Mix well
Place in refrigerator till slightly set
Fold in:
sliced peaches
halved Bing cherries
Return to refrigerator till firm
May be served with plain nonfat yogurt as topping

Estimated nutrition information per serving:

Total fat	0.0 grams	Monounsaturated fat	0.0 grams
Saturated fat	0.0 grams	Polyunsaturated fat	0.0 grams
		Cholesterol	0 milligrams

ORANGE PINEAPPLE GELATIN
serves 6-8

Ingredients:
2 envelopes plain gelatin
$1/2$ cup cold water
$1\ 3/4$ cups orange juice

$1\ 1/2$ cups unsweetened pineapple juice
2 oranges cut in small pieces
1 banana, sliced

Preparation:
Pour into small saucepan:
$1/2$ cup cold water
Sprinkle over water:
2 envelopes gelatin
Heat, stirring constantly till gelatin dissolved
Add:
$1\ 3/4$ cups orange juice
$1\ 1/2$ cups pineapple juice
Mix thoroughly
Pour into bowl
Place in refrigerator till slightly set
Fold in:
orange pieces
1 banana sliced
Return to refrigerator till firm

Estimated nutrition information per serving, $1/8$:

Total fat	0.0 grams	Monounsaturated fat	0.0 grams
Saturated fat	0.0 grams	Polyunsaturated fat	0.0 grams
		Cholesterol	0 milligrams

BANANA & YOGURT
serves 4

Ingredients:

$1/8$ tsp. cinnamon

2 Tbs. concentrated pineapple juice

1 tsp. vanilla

$1/2$ cup plain lowfat yogurt

$1/8$ tsp. nutmeg

4 medium bananas, sliced

Preparation:

Mix together in bowl:

$1/8$ tsp. cinnamon

2 Tbs. concentrated juice

1 tsp. vanilla

$1/2$ cup yogurt

$1/8$ tsp. nutmeg

Fold in:

4 sliced bananas

Chill

Serve topped with sliced fresh fruit if desired

Estimated nutrition information per serving:

Total fat	3 grams	Monounsaturated fat	0.5 grams
Saturated fat	1..4 grams	Polyunsaturated fat	0.1 grams
		Cholesterol	7 milligrams

DANCE STEPS RECIPE

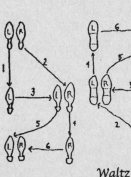

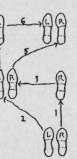

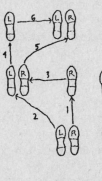

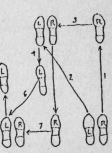

Social Foxtrot

Waltz

BREADS

APPLE OAT BREAD
serves 12

Ingredients:

1 1/2 cups rolled oats
1 1/2 cups whole wheat
   pastry flour
1 1/2 tsp. baking soda
1 1/2 tsp. cinnamon
3/4 tsp. ground allspice

1/4 cup honey
1/2 cup skim milk
3 Tbs. canola oil
3 egg whites
3 med. unpeeled cooking
   apples, diced

Preparation:

Mix together in large bowl:
  1 1/2 cups rolled oats
  1 1/2 cups whole wheat flour
  1 1/2 tsp. baking soda
  1 1/2 tsp. cinnamon
  3/4 tsp. ground allspice
Beat together till blended in small bowl:
  1/4 cup honey
  1/2 cup skim milk
  3 Tbs. oil
  3 egg whites
Stir into flour mixture till flour moistened, will be lumpy
Fold in:
  diced apples
  Spoon into 8 1/2" x 4 1/2" loaf pan sprayed with vegetable
    cooking spray
Bake at 350° 65 minutes or till toothpick inserted into center
  comes out clean.
Cool in pan on wire rack for 10 minutes
Remove from pan
Cool completely on wire rack

Estimated nutrition information per serving:

Total fat	4.6 grams	Monounsaturated fat	2.3 grams
Saturated fat	0.5 grams	Polyunsaturated fat	1.7 grams
		Cholesterol	0 milligrams

OATMEAL RAISIN BREAD
1 loaf

Ingredients:
1 cup whole wheat pastry flour
1 cup rye flour
1 tsp. baking powder
1 tsp. baking soda
1/2 tsp salt

1 cup rolled oats
2 Tbs. molasses
1 2/3 cups plain non fat yogurt
2 tsp. vanilla
1 cup raisins

Preparation:
In bowl mix together with fork:
1 cup whole wheat flour
1 cup rye flour
1 tsp. baking powder
1 tsp. baking soda
$1/2$ tsp. salt
1 cup rolled oats

Beat together in small bowl:
2 Tbs. molasses
1 2/3 cups yogurt
2 tsp. vanilla
Add to dry ingredients
Stir till moistened
Stir in:
1 cup raisins

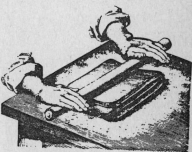

Pour into slightly oiled loaf pan
Let stand 20 minutes

Bake approximately 1 hour at 350°
Delightful with a small amount of low fat cream cheese on a
slice

Estimated nutrition information per serving:

Total fat	5.3 grams	Monounsaturated fat	1.5 grams
Saturated fat	2.7 grams	Polyunsaturated fat	0.5 grams
		Cholesterol	0 milligrams

NO OIL OAT BRAN MUFFINS
12 muffins

Ingredients:

$2^1/4$ cups oat bran

1 Tbs. baking powder

1 Tbs. brown sugar

$1/4$ cup raisins

$1/4$ cup dried apricots, chopped

1 cup nonfat milk

$1/2$ cup orange juice

2 egg whites

$1/4$ cup applesauce

Preparation:

Combine in medium bowl:

$2^1/4$ cups oat bran

1 Tbs. baking powder

1 Tbs. brown sugar

$1/4$ cup raisins

$1/4$ cup chopped apricots

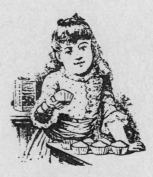

Mix in small bowl:

1 cup milk

$1/2$ cup orange juice

2 egg whites

$1/4$ cup applesauce

Blend with dry ingredients

Pour into paper baking cup lined muffin tins

Bake at 425° for 15 minutes or till inserted pick comes out clean

Remove from pan and serve immediately if desired

Estimated nutrition information per serving:

Total fat	1.3 grams	Monounsaturated fat	0.8 grams
Saturated fat	0.08 grams	Polyunsaturated fat	0.4 grams
		Cholesterol	0.5 milligrams

CORN MUFFINS
10-12 muffins

Ingredients:

$1/3$ cup stirred whole wheat flour

1 tsp. baking powder

$1/4$ tsp. salt

$1/2$ tsp. baking soda

1 Tbs. sugar

$1 \, 1/3$ cups yellow corn meal

1 egg or 2 egg whites, beaten

1 cup lowfat plain yogurt

2 Tbs. canola oil

Preparation:
Stir together in bowl:
$1/3$ cup flour
1 tsp. baking powder
$1/4$ tsp. salt
$1/2$ tsp. baking soda
1 Tbs. sugar
1 $1/3$ cup corn meal

Beat together in small bowl:
egg
1 cup yogurt
2 Tbs. canola oil

Make a well in dry ingredients
Add yogurt mixture
Stir till just blended
Pour into oiled muffin tins

Bake at 400° for 25 minutes

Estimated nutrition information per serving: (made with 1 whole egg)

Total fat	3.4 grams	Monounsaturated fat	1.7 grams
Saturated fat	0.5 grams	Polyunsaturated fat	1.0 grams
		Cholesterol	20 milligrams

ZUCCHINI MUFFIN
8 muffins

Ingredients:

$3/4$ cup whole wheat pastry flour
$3/4$ tsp. baking powder
$3/4$ tsp. cinnamon
$1/4$ tsp. nutmeg
$1/2$ tsp. baking soda
$1/8$ tsp. salt

$1/2$ tsp. vanilla extract
2 Tbs. concentrated orange juice
1 Tbs. canola oil
4 egg whites
1 cup shredded, unpeeled zucchini
$1/3$ cup raisins

Preparation:
Combine in small bowl:
$3/4$ cup flour
$3/4$ tsp. baking powder
$3/4$ tsp. cinnamon
$1/4$ tsp. nutmeg
$1/2$ tsp. baking soda
$1/8$ tsp. salt
Mix well with fork

Combine in large bowl:
$1/2$ tsp. vanilla
2 Tbs. concentrated orange juice
1 Tbs. oil
4 egg whites
Beat on low speed of mixer till blended

Add:
dry ingredients
Beat on low speed until all ingredients just moistened
Stir in:
1 cup zucchini
$1/3$ cup raisins

Spoon into 8 nonstick muffin tins
Bake 15-17 minutes at 350°
Cool 10 minutes before removing from tins

Estimated nutrition information per serving:

Total fat	2.1 grams	Monounsaturated fat	1.0 grams
Saturated fat	0.2 grams	Polyunsaturated fat	0.8 grams
		Cholesterol	0 milligrams

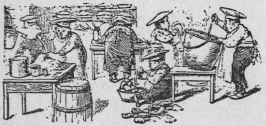

Handbook Index

ORDER YOUR COPY(S) TODAY!

_____ copy(s) **THE LOW BLOOD SUGAR HANDBOOK** $12.95

_____ copy(s) **THE LOW BLOOD SUGAR COOKBOOK** $12.95

_____ _ copy(s) **THE LOW BLOOD SUGAR CASSETTE (1 HOUR)** $9.95

_____ copy(s) **VITAL HEALTH FACTS & composition of foods charts** . $4.50

_____ copy(s) **CHOLESTEROL CONTROL 3 WEEK PLAN: HANDBOOK &
COOKBOOK** .... $15..95

Send note or copy of order form with payment

Send check or postal money order to: Franklin Publishers, Box 1338, Bryn Mawr,
PA 19010. **U.S. orders** add postage of $2 for 1 item, $3 for 2 items, $4 for 3 or
more items. **PA residents** add state sales tax. **Canadian orders** add postage of $3
for 1 item, $4 for 2 items, $5 for 3 or more items. **All other countries** add postage
of $7 for 1 item, $10 for 2 items, $13 for 3 or more items. **All orders outside U.S.**
must be paid in U.S. Dollars by postal money order.

Send to: Mr/Ms._____

Address_____

City _____State_____Zip_____

Phone number _____

Price subject to change without notice

ORDER YOUR COPY(S) TODAY!

_____ copy(s) **THE LOW BLOOD SUGAR HANDBOOK** $12.95

_____ copy(s) **THE LOW BLOOD SUGAR COOKBOOK** $12.95

_____ _ copy(s) **THE LOW BLOOD SUGAR CASSETTE (1 HOUR)** $9.95

_____ copy(s) **VITAL HEALTH FACTS & composition of foods charts** . $4.50

_____ copy(s) **CHOLESTEROL CONTROL 3 WEEK PLAN: HANDBOOK &
COOKBOOK** $15.95

Send note or copy of order form with payment

Send check or postal money order to: Franklin Publishers, Box 1338, Bryn Mawr,
PA 19010. **U.S. orders** add postage of $2 for 1 item, $3 for 2 items, $4 for 3 or
more items. **PA residents** add state sales tax. **Canadian orders** add postage of $3
for 1 item, $4 for 2 items, $5 for 3 or more items. **All other countries** add postage
of $7 for 1 item, $10 for 2 items, $13 for 3 or more items. **All orders outside U.S.**
must be paid in U.S. Dollars by postal money order.

Send to: Mr/Ms._____

Address_____

City _____State_____Zip_____

Phone number _____

ORDER YOUR COPY(S) TODAY!

_____ copy(s)   **THE LOW BLOOD SUGAR HANDBOOK** $12.95

_____ copy(s)   **THE LOW BLOOD SUGAR COOKBOOK** $12.95

_____ copy(s)   **THE LOW BLOOD SUGAR CASSETTE (1 HOUR)** $9.95

_____ copy(s)   **VITAL HEALTH FACTS & composition of foods charts** . $4.50

_____ copy(s)   **CHOLESTEROL CONTROL 3 WEEK PLAN: HANDBOOK &**
                   COOKBOOK $15.95

Send note or copy of order form with payment

Send check or postal money order to: Franklin Publishers, Box 1338, Bryn Mawr, PA 19010. **U.S. orders** add postage of $2 for 1 item, $3 for 2 items, $4 for 3 or more items. **PA residents** add state sales tax. **Canadian orders** add postage of $3 for 1 item, $4 for 2 items, $5 for 3 or more items. **All other countries** add postage of $7 for 1 item, $10 for 2 items, $13 for 3 or more items. **All orders outside U.S.** must be paid in U.S. Dollars by postal money order.

Send to: Mr/Ms._____

Address_____

City _____ State_____ Zip_____

Phone number _____

Price subject to change without notice

ORDER YOUR COPY(S) TODAY!

_____ copy(s)   **THE LOW BLOOD SUGAR HANDBOOK** $12.95

_____ copy(s)   **THE LOW BLOOD SUGAR COOKBOOK** $12.95

_____ copy(s)   **THE LOW BLOOD SUGAR CASSETTE (1 HOUR)** $9.95

_____ copy(s)   **VITAL HEALTH FACTS & composition of foods charts** . $4.50

_____ copy(s)   **CHOLESTEROL CONTROL 3 WEEK PLAN: HANDBOOK &**
                   COOKBOOK $15.95

Send note or copy of order form with payment

Send check or postal money order to: Franklin Publishers, Box 1338, Bryn Mawr, PA 19010. **U.S. orders** add postage of $2 for 1 item, $3 for 2 items, $4 for 3 or more items. **PA residents** add state sales tax. **Canadian orders** add postage of $3 for 1 item, $4 for 2 items, $5 for 3 or more items. **All other countries** add postage of $7 for 1 item, $10 for 2 items, $13 for 3 or more items. **All orders outside U.S.** must be paid in U.S. Dollars by postal money order.

Send to: Mr/Ms._____

Address_____

City _____ State_____ Zip_____

Phone number _____

Patricia and Edward Krimmel are medical writers who have a special aptitude and spirit for relating well to those trying to solve health problems. Because of their backgrounds, they are especially well prepared to write and design books dealing with solutions rather than simply talking about the problems.

Pat and Ed are known nationally within personal health care circles as true "authorities." They are the authors of two best sellers; The Low Blood Sugar Handbook and The Low Blood Sugar Cookbook. They are frequent guests on radio and television shows from coast to coast and give lectures at health seminars.

Pat has her BSN from the University of Pennsylvania, has worked in childbirth education (CEA) and public health and has been maternal and infant care coordinator at the Medical College of Pennsylvania.

Ed has his degree in Social Science from St. Joseph's University, is director of HELP, The Institute for Body Chemistry, and does nutritional counseling.

David M. Capuzzi, M.D., Ph.D. is Director of the Cardiovascular Disease Prevention Center, Director of the Center's Lipoprotein - Atherosclerosis Laboratory, and Professor of Medicine, Biochemistry, and Molecular Pharmacology, Thomas Jefferson University, Philadelphia, Pennsylvania. He is attending Physician in Endocrinology, Diabetes, Metabolism, and Preventive Cardiology at the Thomas Jefferson University Hospital, and Consulting Physician in diabetes and Endocrinology at the Lankenau Hospital, Wynnewood, Pennsylvania.

The primary goal of his Centers' work is the prevention of initial or recurrent heart attack or stroke that results from the buildup of fatty plagues (atherosclerosis) in the inner lining of major arteries. Treatment is directed toward correcting the abnormalities in lipoprotein metabolism that cause atherosclerosis. Dr. Capuzzi and his coworkers have conducted many research studies in this field, and have documented their finding in numerous scientific articles.